An injunction of a Mayfair hairdresser

James Dillon

 New Generation **Publishing**

As with most children at the age of sixteen, I too was urging myself ever nearer to the end of my school years. To be honest, I never really liked school. I wasn't the most popular kid, although neither was I the most unpopular kid in my year. Let's say more of the average student.

I didn't dislike the teachers or the other pupils, I guess I just didn't like the thought of knowing that I had to go to school every single day. There really was no other excuse.

I can always remember my parents telling me that their school days were always the best days of their lives, but I can assure you they certainly weren't mine. I also remember them telling me once that if I didn't go to school that they themselves would be sent to prison. I am sure looking back that this was a last ditch attempt to get me to go to school when I hid myself under the bed on the occasional morning. It didn't really matter to me whether what they said was either true or false it made me go, and to this day I must thank them as they were doing what all good parents should.

When we are younger we never like to admit that our parents are right, however as we get older we begin to realize that unfortunately most of the time our parents are right and within time we grow to be just like them.

Both my parents were in full time work, well, my father was a welding engineer and electrician running his own business and my mother a full time mum. I say the word full time as looking after two energetic sons myself and my older brother I think it's safe to say that they were both definitely full time parents. We were not the easiest of boys to control as far as young boys go.

My father had a factory outside of town and in the summer holidays I used to spend a lot of time going to work with him. Not only did I go to the factory for something to do during the holidays I also enjoyed spending time with my dad, after all, all parents are your hero's when you are young, you always feel untouchable, never have to pay for anything (including taxis) and you never feel that you have any problems when they are around, Well, apart from the odd 'I hate you' moment from time to time.

I loved going to work with my dad, I would like to say I loved helping him at work but I guess I never really helped him that much, I think I got in the way more than anything. I suppose he had to give me something to do to keep me occupied throughout the day so he could get on with doing some serious work and so I was given small tasks to do like dismantling things such as broken welding machines, stripping dirty cables or pretending to fix fans which I knew nothing about. If they weren't really broken already they pretty much were when I had finished with them. I also cleaned machines that where oily and greasy trying to make them look like new again, however as I look back they were all still caked up with dust and oil although it had kept me quiet and out of his way for at lease twenty minutes or so. I enjoyed doing all these odd, useless jobs and that was all that mattered at the time.

It was around the age of thirteen that I knew for sure that getting my hands dirty, cut, oily or greasy was not my kind of thing, nothing of course to do with having to take a bath everyday, another thing that as a child never seemed that important. As I have grown up and looked back I have learnt so much from my father. At times when I never looked interested or seemed as though I was never listening there were many times I learnt something new, fun and educational.

As both myself and my brother got older and went to school my mum went back to work part time at a leisure centre in a crèche looking after toddlers while their parents were working hard to provide for their own household, and also for people like my mum to look after their children. Nowadays it sometimes seems we have less and less time for our children whether or not we have become more self absorbed or selfish in our own interests, or whether work is becoming more and more demanding, you decide ?

Going to work with my mum unfortunately wasn't as much fun as work with my dad, I think it was more because I was at the teenage stage myself and kids where defiantly not on my agenda as playing in play doe and sandpits was so not cool. It wasn't all bad however, going for lunch with my mum was great, fish and chips or a chip butty was always worth waiting for on the way home in the local pub.

I think as I've become older my wise attributes have come from my dad and a softer, sincere side has come from my mum, I wouldn't want it any other way.

And so at sixteen with no real GCSE's and the idea of having great aspirations of becoming a hairstylist, I knew then it wasn't really something to shout about the least impressive or the most manly idea a sixteen year old boy could tell his mates that he was wanting to be when he left school, especially growing up in Derbyshire where as most of the jobs at the time were things like factory work, plumbing, electrician, painting and decorating, mechanics and general getting your hands dirty kind of work, mans work they call it !

It all began with work experience. I think to be fair, I did put down three things that I wanted to have a go at, three things that included all of those manly jobs but unfortunately my school couldn't find me a placement at the time. Honestly that's the truth. And so as a last resort I kind of said "hairdressing" and that was it, within a few days they found me a placement in a small local salon in town.

The town I lived in was a very small town called Ripley in Derbyshire. For anyone who hasn't been to Ripley let me give you a quick brief, number one, Ripley is a pretty small town and apart from the usual things like having a sports centre, library, pharmacy and shops, not forgetting Ripley does have a town hall, it is also filled with pubs, clubs and take-aways in which people spill out of every Friday and Saturday night, but don't be put off by this because Ripley has actually been named the most English/British town in the UK today. So there you have it....Ripley in a nutshell.

There is also a Ripley in Yorkshire and the only reason I know this is because our post was sometimes late getting to us as it had been sent to the wrong Ripley, so there.

I remember the Friday I finished school and met my mum in town to go and buy some new trousers and a new shirt ready for my first day of my work experience at the salon. I always remember meeting her in town as it wasn't cool if it was your mum standing waiting at the school gates for you when the school bell had rang for home time. It was embarrassing. It was always a rule at school between your friends to never ever let your parents meet you at the school gates, other kids could see them through the window while they were still in lessons knowing that they was going to tell at least one person next to them in class who's mother or father it was, and then once established who's parent it was it would then go around the whole class like Chinese whispers and that poor child would look an idiot, just as if they weren't allowed to walk home on their own like other kids.

I was no different, I didn't want to be picked on or made to be the laughing stock so it was safe to say I decided to meet my mum in town away from any of my mates.

Now, I don't know what it is with mums, I can understand they are proud of their children and always want you to look your best, but why do they insist in always dressing you like a cardboard cut out? Things that you like are not always what they like and what they like is so not fashionable and the shops that you like are cool, trendy and maybe a little more expensive than what they have in mind, so as you can guess, it was mums choice of shop and mums choice of clothes. I tried so desperately hard to tempt my mum in taking me to the shops I wanted but you get to a stage of arguing when you just know when to shut up and keep quiet.

Everything I tried on was either too tight or too long but hey guess what? Mum liked it! I can understand the concept of smart, but the idea of black trousers black shirt and black shoes with bright red hair was not my idea of "wow" I love it, when really the only thought that was running through my head was "all the girls in this salon are going to think I've been dressed by my mother and what a Pratt!"

In the end we both opted for a dark blue checkered shirt (which I really liked) and black trousers so we both had our input and we were both happy, kind of anyway.

Thanks mum.

I woke early Monday morning excited about my first day of my work experience.

I never really ate breakfast, neither did I have a hot drink before I left the house, but today my dad insisted.

He always told myself and my brother never to leave the house in the morning without having something to eat and drink, "it's the most important meal of the day" he used to say, it was like his ritual, however seeing my dad eating two slices of toast smothered in thick dripping wasn't something that I looked forward too as much as he did the night before.

He was Derbyshire born and Derbyshire bred as they say. In my opinion bread and dripping should have been made illegal it was dreadful stuff, surely, its just pure lard?

While I'm on the subject here are a few foods that I think should also be made illegal, cod liver oil, lard, black pudding, semolina and rice pudding. In my mind these are all evil foods and may I just say that these are also foods our parents told us were good for you. So you have been warned.

The salon was in the centre of town and was within walking distance from our house. That morning when I left home I remember feeling really good about myself, almost proud, in fact, I felt so good that the goodness in me took over all of my nerves, I already felt like I knew what I was letting myself in for. After all, I looked good, I had made an effort with my hair and I had all new clothes, I was looking good and feeling good what else did I need?

It was only until I caught the salon in sight that I started to have my doubts, I started to walk slower and slower but somehow I was nearing the salon much quicker than I had intended. I was already early so to pass some time I walked the circumference of the market place as not to look too eager, too ready or too much of a goody goody for turning up way too on time even though my freshly straightened hair was starting to curl up and frizz in the light drizzle of rain blanketing down from the depressing grey sky.

Walking around the market square didn't help. It gave me more time to think and more time to worry about things.

I looked at my watch time and time again trying to judge the right time to start my beeline to the salon and also until my hair couldn't take much more of the damp weather.

As I walked up to the salon door I was becoming more and more restless, my hands and my forehead were becoming sweaty and I was running through my mind all the things I was going to say to whoever I met once I was in the salon, whether it be a receptionist or manager or any one I bumped in to. I was beginning to stress.
I reached the door.

I took a few long deep breaths and pushed open the worn, varnished wooden door entering an environment unknown to me, however, once opened my heart sank reality kicked in and I had lost all feeling of self control and confidence.

I had now come face to face with being out of my comfort zone.

In front of me was a stair case. I know it doesn't

sound very scary, but when you're expecting to be greeted by another human resembling a form of receptionist and instead a set of stairs, I was at this point panicking. This wasn't what I was expecting so soon had I entered the salon, come to think of it I wasn't actually in the salon yet.

At the bottom of the stair case the salon seemed quiet, no music and no talking just a green carpet of about fifteen steps, to the left of me was an oval shaped mirror in which I wiped away the beads of sweat from my forehead and tampered with my hair trying not to look so vain just in case any one did see me or there were cameras around watching me.

I slowly walked up the stairs holding on to the wooded hand rail telling myself there was nothing to worry about when all I could do was think the opposite. What was wrong with me? Ten minutes ago I was so confidant I could take on the whole of Ripley, and now I was like a child again at my first day of school, not knowing where to go or what to do.

At the top of the stairs on the left was a solid wooden door, it was still very quiet and not a sound of any hairdryers or the smell of perm lotion which is always a smell you remember even if you've only stood foot in a hair salon once in your life. I opened the door with a nervous almost pathetic push from the palm of my sweaty hand and in front of me was the reception and one woman whom I was assuming was the receptionist. I calmly introduced myself. She was nice, a little on the larger scale than I had expected but she was nice. (Later, I grew to like this woman very much).

I waited while she made a phone call and within seconds word had reached the staff room of my arrival and a stream of girls quickly came flowing in to the reception area to introduce themselves and to have a nosey at who they had working with them for the rest of the week. It was just like I was an alien to them, although very polite and equally nice I was the centre of attention, I was feeling like I was being examined poked at and prodded, then again, it seemed I was the only male in the salon. I was like the new boy.

I was introduced to all the girls and shown around the salon, you know, all the do's and don'ts, being shown the ropes and all that and then it was time for the first arrivals of clients to come in for their appointments.

The salon was small yet cozy no special mirrors or chairs just the basics. Basins to wash hair and shelving with rollers gathering dust, the kind of rollers you tend to see in old ladies hair, the kind of purple rinse and old time sets. Towels were neatly folded on shelves symmetrically and products were being advertised in military style displays around the salon. It was very nice and simple and very disciplined.

It was a novelty at first being the new boy of the salon especially with the conversations between the stylist and the clients talking about me as if I wasn't even in the same environment as they were, I suppose it was different for the clients as well, whispering and smirking looking at me not directly but through the mirrors. They were good, they were very good, the stylists worked at the salon every day year after year and they knew which mirrors they could look through to see whatever part of the salon they wanted without being noticed by any one else, but hey I wasn't stupid, I soon clocked on to knowing the sequence as to where wandering eyes patrolled and found myself learning their trait which would become useful later in time.

It didn't take long until I was doing it so often myself I became a pro, it also passed a little time during the day.

The first day in the salon I was kind of left to observing the salon environment, the odd stylist spoke to me and asked me from time to time if I was ok and if I was enjoying the day so far? However, others didn't say a thing to me, these were mainly the juniors.

Juniors were basically skivvies that did all the shitty work like make cups of coffee but not just for the clients, that would be understandable, but for the stylists or clean the salon or staff room not just for the clients sake but because the stylist didn't seem to be able to clean up their own mess, and also tidying the staff room, you guessed it, not after yourself but for the stylists who left their rubbish from their lunch on the floor or tables and for some reason couldn't reach the bins, "this is it " I thought, to become a hairdresser I need to get through this. I quickly learnt to clean and tidy emptying bins and tidying magazines, hovering and wiping things down with damp cloths. And so that was that, I had now become a self confessed skivvy junior.

As I was growing up I was always taught right from wrong and even though in my teenage years I became more and more opinionated and strong minded I had to remember I was here to learn and do what I was told, and most importantly set a good example of how capable I was in this profession, even if I'd never ever picked up a pair of scissors or a comb before. Yes I could clean and yes I could make tea and coffee and sweep up but I hadn't expected to carry others, especially the juniors. I had the feeling because I was new I was relied upon by the juniors to do most of the work that they should have been doing themselves, but after all, I was new and had to get on with it.

During the week experience it became second nature of doing the whole series of tasks from cleaning and preparing to towel rosters and client care, I also learnt where to be at what time and what to do when. I never needed to be asked or told to do anything, I was on the ball, always thinking ahead and always being ever ready for everything and everyone, but within time it was made very clear to me by the juniors that trying to impress my peers wasn't the way the juniors liked you to be, there seemed to be a role, a ranking if you like and I was at the bottom of it. The juniors didn't seem to like anyone enthusiastic or liked by the stylists, it was clear a jealous state had set in and it was only the beginning of things to come.

I found it hard to get in to my head that the

juniors didn't like me since I had tried so hard to try and fit in. I did all the dirty work for them. I put out the bins, disinfected the bathrooms, washed the towels and cleaned the staffroom but because I wanted to come across as capable, especially to the manager. I also tried not to work as hard just so I would be liked and accepted by the juniors themselves.

There seemed to be a game to play in this profession and I certainly hadn't played this game before.

This week followed every day pretty much the same throughout apart from the fact that most of my mates had started texting me regarding what I was doing for my weeks work experience. I just knew I couldn't tell them the truth that I seriously wanted to become a hairdresser and a straight one at that! I had to make up excuses of being busy at the local mechanics garage and that I didn't get a lunch break because I was always so busy but the excuses were running thin especially when it came to them wanting to meet up after work for a catch up.

I enjoyed what I was doing and I loved getting up in the morning with the feeling of going to work and that was something I never thought I would say but I did, I enjoyed every minute of it and that was part of my problem with the juniors, the only person I really got on with was the salon owner and the receptionist, however I found myself separating myself further and further away from them just so I fitted in with the juniors.

I used to think wow this beats going to school

any day after hearing all those times by your parents, aunties and uncles going on about how school was the best days of their lives and make the most of it…yeah right, or the most famous line of all which was 'your only young once'!!!! I think you forget all these sayings until you reach a certain age and then when you hit that time period in your life you find yourself saying the same things that your parents did and you then pass them down to your own kids or somebody else's who equally find it either boring or a load of shit.

I can remember it was a Friday as it was my last day of my work experience at the salon but it may as well have been the 13th just to top off my week. I was feeling confidant that I had found a job that I really enjoyed, it was busy yet it was also laid back at the same time and at the end of the day when the salon was tidy and all the towels had been washed and put out to dry it was my turn to have a go at learning the art of shampooing a head of hair. The lucky victim was the manager's last client of the day. I'm not sure if I was meant to say lucky or actually, unlucky.

I stood at the side of the back wash watching intensely and listening nervously at the instructions I was being given by the manager, she did the first shampoo and I did the second being as careful as possible to get my technique right. It was almost embarrassing, me, a guy trying to shampoo, what would my mates think or say if they could see me now? There was a slight element of femininity about the whole process of mixing flowing strokes and firm pressure and trying my best at physiologically pleasing the client with only the use of my mind and hands even though my mind was really thinking about how attractive I found my boss and not fucking up this supposedly luxury shampoo.

I probably tried too hard to impress, I just wanted so much to get it right that even the way I leant over the basin and stood looked slightly awkward but I tried my best and in a weird way it felt kind of nice, I'm sorry but it did, I'm not being gay or anything but it did and for anyone who still finds it weird then try it sometime as it may bring out a different side to you that you never thought you had. Therapeutic is the word.

We conditioned the clients hair massaging the scalp at all times and rinsing with delicacy making sure not to wet the client or remove any make up from her forehead. I also learnt the art of wrapping a towel around the head in such a way that when the client stood up it made her look like she had Mickey mouse ears which kind of helped create a giggle between us all and took off a little pressure from myself, even though it was probably the worst shampoo this client had ever had, however, she told me it was very nice and I could do it again on her next visit but I'm sure she was just a very good liar and had already made her mind up on which other salon she could go to next time if I ever got a job at this particular salon.

Before I packed my belongings in to my school bag I said my thank you's and goodbyes and all the other things you say to make you sound like you really enjoyed every minute of every day even though there had been moments that were not all that great and I finally got my chance to say thank you to the manager for having me. I liked her, she had a friendly persona about her which made many of the staff and clients warm to her. She always made me feel welcome.

She told me it had been a real pleasure and one day in the week I was to call in after school to say hello to everyone and so she could chat to me regarding a job opportunity. As excited as I was I hid it until I was out of the salon, after all I think with me being the only male in the salon it was not only a novelty but it was exciting for the other female stylists to have me around if I don't mind saying so myself.

As I walked home that evening I caught glimpses of myself in the shop windows smirking at myself at the fact I had shampooed my first ever client as if I was the best shampooer in the history of the hairdressing world and if there was any competitions or awards in shampooing then I would be nominated, not exactly taking in to account that the juniors were skilled professionals in this and they were doing around at least ten shampoos every day to my one in a week. They had been trained and shown the ropes long before I arrived but I knew I could learn fast and I could be up there on par with them.

I couldn't wait to get home and tell my mum how my day had been or that I could end up with a job.

I didn't want to jump the gun but I was already thinking about how the hell I could get out of going back to school or doing my exams, at the end of the day who needs grades when I had found the job of a lifetime? I was excitingly talking to myself walking through the park on the way home when my mobile phone made the sound of a received text, I quickly scurried around in my pockets to find my phone, it was one of my friends, I thought before I had even read the message that it would probably be about meeting up for drinks later that evening, and after the week I had I was damn sure I was going to be going out.

Even though I wasn't old enough to drink there was always a certain pub you knew that would never ask you for your identification and because of that it was always classed as your very own local, however, instead of it being a text regarding a drink it was quiet the opposite, it was one of those moments when you just wished the floor would open up and you would sink beneath it, or even better, you was moving to a far away place where nobody knew you and you would never bump in to any one you knew ever again.

The text read as follows, "My mum said you've just washed her hair"!!!

Well I was devastated, there was no longer an excuse or a comment I could think of to send back via a text, I say text because there was no way I was going to pick up the phone and have a half hour chat with him about how fabulous my week had been in a local hair salon, meeting and greeting clients, chatting away about holidays and the weather and the usual talk you tend to find in most salons, along with "are you doing anything nice today"? and all that spiel, especially when he'd been working like a real man making window frames in a factory were men were men, the kind of men that went to the gym every night pumped with steroids and then sank around fourteen pints of lager in the evenings or at least every other night, the men who went out for all hours at night and still seemed to have the time to get up and make a packed lunch for work before they left the house, strong useful men. And then there was me, a poxy hairdresser well not even a hairdresser, a junior or skiv at that. Me, who would have to make tea and coffee in between rubbing on hand cream to protect my sore hands from chapping whilst waiting for the kettle to boil.

I didn't reply straight back as you can imagine I had to take a little time thinking about what I was going to say and after a few moments of sheer embarrassment I plucked up the courage and found myself explaining my piece about the real job prospect I had chosen and why. After all, there were no problems after meeting up in the local for a few beers later and a huge amount of piss taking. Once it was all said and done life carried on pretty normal. At the end of the day mates are mates through thick and thin and if you can't laugh at your self then who can you laugh at, eh?

Although my friends and family respected the fact that I wanted to do hairdressing there always seemed to be a problem with my friend's parents, it was the parents who I mainly had a hard time with. Whenever I went round to see my friends and their parents were in they would always seem to bring up the whole "what are you going to do when you leave school"?

To which I replied "hairdressing"

I got the whole low down on how there was no money to be made in hairdressing and that how much more clever and bright I was and should consider doing something that would pay more and was more intellectual, it was just as if they already knew everything about the hair industry like they all had been there and done it, but I was adamant I knew what I wanted to do and the more I heard people tell me not to do it the more I wanted to succeed and prove I could do it, so I just smiled and tried to change the conversation to anything not to do with working in hairdressing.

The weekend was the same old usual, steady, nothing to stressful weekend.

Mum and dad were up and had gone out doing their thing as they always did.

Parents always have the idea that a lie in was until around 8.30am, why do parents always think its normal to get up early? Even on a Sunday. Why do they feel the need to have breakfast and walk to the shop for the Sunday newspaper so early? Why? The printers print loads of this shit every weekend.

The weekend for me was the slowest on record, the only thing on my mind was getting out of school on time so I could get back to the salon and see the manager to discuss whether or not I might just have a job when I left school.

After all the times of getting out of bed and going to school when I didn't want to I was almost wishing my life away, almost wanting to go back to school so I could find out about this job.

Monday had slowly come around and today I was ready to get up and go to school in the hope that the sooner I got there the sooner the day would end.

I found myself watching the clocks in every lesson wishing I had a super power of some kind that could take off a few hours or fast forward the clocks to half past four.

I don't know what it is, but people do say that when your enjoying something time seems to go really quickly and when your not enjoying something then it can drag, well, how true that it, my day went so slow. I couldn't concentrate on my lessons during the day, my mind just kept on playing back footage of the days I was doing my work experience but as soon as the end of the day bell rang I was out that school and heading in to town towards the salon.

I walked quickly to the salon cutting through allotments and hedges to gain time. My shins were aching with rushing so much so that I am surprised I didn't give myself shin splinters.

As I reached the salon once again I had become nervous but equally excited about pushing open the door walking up the stairs and opening the door to the reception, it was just like my first day all over again.

I was greeted by the receptionist and I walked around the salon to the other stylists to say hi. It must have been a good sign as they all seemed really happy to see me, the only people who didn't seem happy nor did they approach me and say hi was the juniors, but I guess I didn't expect them to, at the end of the day I was here for my benefit and not theirs.

The salon was busy, hairdryers blowing and stylist chatting away to their clients along with music playing in the background. I wanted to stay and be part of the team but I knew I was here to see the manager and find out if this was going to be a reality or I was going to be in for the biggest let down of my life.

I sat patiently on the sofa in the reception whilst the manager was finishing her client my eyes wandering around the salon walls interior.

Soon the manager had finished her client and we walked down the corridor to the staff room the door closed behind. It was suddenly quiet, no noise from the hairdryers and no business from the salon floor. It was just myself and her which slightly caused me to panic as I expected the worst. I expected I was going to be let down as gently as possible and that there actually wasn't a position for me at the salon.

We sat at a table opposite each other in silence so to break the ice I came up with the most cringe worthy line you could ever imagine as if I was sixteen going on thirty, "Been busy today"? That was the best I could do.

She asked me how my day was and if I had enjoyed my weeks work experience to which I answered. We were both all smiles but all I could think about was why is she being so nice and polite to me if I'm going to hear the words of we haven't got a position for you here. The tension was building and I was waiting for the negatives, it was like waiting to be hung.

The time had come and this was it, time for the words I was dreading, time to start putting my head through the noose, but it wasn't what I was expecting, the words "when can you start"? echoed through my ears I felt like I had just won the lottery, a feeling that I'd never feel as I have never played the lottery but from now on there would be no more worries, not only had I got a job but I couldn't wait to tell my parents, they would be so happy for me.

I think parents like to think that one day comes along where you, their children, make them feel proud and I thought that this was that moment but later on there was much more to come to which none of us where to know what was around the corner.

My parents were ecstatic when I told them and every family member soon got to know I had got a job in hairdressing. When we went to visit my aunties and uncles my new job seemed to be the main point of conversation and how well I'd done, so much so it became embarrassing. That's parents and family for you!

As soon as I'd finished sitting my exams I started work as a full time apprentice junior in the salon. I attended model evenings after work where I practiced the art of shampooing and blow-drying, I also attended college once a week in the beginning which increased to once a month as I worked up the ladder from blow-drying to perming and setting hair and then the cutting side of things.

I seemed to pick up on things very quickly and never had to be told twice, I enjoyed the work and nothing was a problem, I always knew that the days were going to be long with many late nights along with the sore hands from the constant shampooing (especially over the Christmas period) however, I also noticed I was doing more work than most of the other juniors, they seemed to get out of doing most of the work especially the shampoos because they themselves didn't want to get sore hands. It seemed as though they always got out of doing the work but always accepted the praise for tidying the staffroom, bathrooms or washing up etc, when really it was me who just seemed to get on with the chores, but hey, who was I to say anything? At the end of the day I was the new kid, I couldn't just say what I thought and voice my opinions. It was still early days and I didn't want to get in to any trouble.

I tried to get on with the other juniors the best I could but unfortunately to no avail. It was hard to find a connection with them as the juniors would go out at the weekends together and go shopping or meet up for social gatherings, I was a guy and I guess I was just made to feel different. Trying hard to be friends just wasn't going to happen.

Within time whilst working at the salon I was hearing requests from clients wanting me to shampoo their hair when they visited the salon and the odd blow-dry here and there, luckily the manager let me do it but the more positive the comments I received from clients the worst it became with myself and the juniors, a jealousy had built up for such a long time it was slowly starting to get to me and upset me. There was nothing that I could say to anyone in the salon about the way I felt because when you work in a salon you soon get to realize that no secrets can be kept between the staff even if it 'IS' a private matter, gossip is the one thing that most hairdressers are good at and I felt enclosed.

Every so often we would have staff meetings bringing up points of interests from the stylists. They were held on the salon floor after working hours and the more meetings we had the more topics where being headed towards myself. I never really had anything to say in the meetings, the reason being was because I felt that as I was the only male sat between ten women it always made me feel like I was going to be ganged up on and so it was very seldom that I spoke about any issues that I had. I tended to just to sit and look at the floor.

I was so in to my work that every time something negative was pointed towards being my fault I just wanted to try and improve on being better and better at working towards becoming a great stylist.

Things were beginning to change and not for the better.

The bullying came shortly after, I found it harder and harder to get up in the morning to go to work, and I knew that it wasn't like me to not want to go in but the bullying was holding me back, why couldn't I say anything? And why did nobody else seem to see it?

It took me a long time to realize I had it in me to start finding some backbone, I really couldn't take it anymore. I spent days going through in my head what I wanted the manager to know and what I wanted everyone to be aware of and how it was making me feel.

Many nights as I walked home from the salon I would take the time to sit in the local park and have a little cry to myself while I practiced how and what I wanted to say to my manager without feeling I was going to get myself or anyone else in to trouble.

Then one day, I decided that the time had come for me to pluck up the courage and say my piece in the next staff meeting.

We all sat in a circle facing each other every body in the same chairs in the same position as always looking tired after a long day at work, well, for some. The meeting started and the topics were in full flow. There were three kind of stylists in this salon, firstly, there were the kind of stylists that liked to say their piece and get things off their chest, these stylists seemed to be the sensible types and generally wanted the best for the salon, then came the stylists that didn't really have anything of any decency to talk about but would agree on anything that the manager thought was a good or bad idea, when really these stylists just liked to hear the slight squeak's of their own voice. I guess you find this in every business and office through out every company around the world.

And then you get the ones that have a huge amount to say during the salons working day although when it comes to meetings all of a sudden they have nothing to say at all, and everything in their books is ok and they were happy with everything. In reality all they really wanted to do was go home as they really didn't care. These were mainly the juniors that for months and months had given me a hard time.

The time came when it was up to me to say anything that I thought needed to be brought in to the meeting and so with a deep breath I said what I had to say.

All hell broke loose from the first sentence, from a calm, cool meeting to a sudden rise in temperatures around the room, you could actually see the heat as a redness started to climb up people's necks and on to their faces. It was a long awaited meeting which had been building up for quiet some time.

The language was unbearable and there was a lot of shouting bringing rage and a moment of madness, where it seemed as though every one at one point had something to say. Stylists were talking over one another not being able to understand each others opinions.

Once a structure had been strictly put in place by the manager the meeting was brought to a swift end and we were all dismissed, however I could sense it had left a slightly dissatisfied reaction from many and we all retired home.

I hadn't meant for the meeting to end this way although I had said my piece, unfortunately, I felt I had caused a huge unsettlement with in the team spirit.

After this meeting the days that followed were never the same, as much as every body tried to get on there was always a kind of awkwardness from time to time but never was anything ever discussed with myself about the meeting from the manager or the other stylists.

I found it hard to work there and the enjoyment was slowly and surely fizzling out, I didn't enjoy the training side of things either, I had lost interest in the working environment, the days dragged and I felt like know one cared about the way I felt. Part of me felt like I was the one to blame, if only I had kept my mouth closed none of this would have happened although I felt I had also been singled out from the very start, I'd been bullied and treated like an individual segregated from being friends with others friends. I felt like I was in a constant battle I had already lost. I couldn't believe all the things I had done, my attendance was second to none and everything I was told to do I did, after all the energy I gave I couldn't accept the way I was being treated, it was as if everyone wanted to forget about it all rather than deal with the problems that were occurring.

My work ethic was crumbling and my smile had been noticeably lost. I used to speak to my parents about the problems but my parents kept telling me to stick it out until I was qualified but all I wanted to do was get out of the work place as soon as I could, I couldn't wait to get home, who'd of thought I used to be so enthusiastic and outgoing when I first started working in the salon from the days of arriving early to now not wanting to even be there.

It was whilst I was doing my exams at school that I chose to do my revision at home. I'm not sure I actually did any revision as I can always remember watching a lot of television on those so called revision days. I used to constantly flick through the channels. It didn't take me long to channel hop as at the time my parents had one of those huge TV's, the ones with a big back, you know the ones I'm talking about, they only had five channels. I can remember going up and down the channels until I ended up watching breakfast TV.

Its content was predictable. The soap obsessive who knew what we should all be expecting to see on the screens for the coming weeks and the agony aunt who tried to help with viewers problems. It always made me laugh to think that all these people whilst on TV may come across as very professional but in real life I often thought they could have been married three times before themselves, possibly with children from different men or women and a nasty drink problem that if it wasn't for finding god they would have never of got through it. These people always seemed to have been there and done it and were now trying to advise others on how to cope.

I don't know if you've ever noticed but there is always an interview with someone who has dropped from a size twenty to a size eight in less than five months, big deal, why don't they have people on these shows who make huge differences in the world or even the community? I reckon I could get an OBE just for work ethic nowadays.

But amongst all this was a morning make over. This is when they find somebody who really deserves a makeover (or has terrible hair, and I mean TERRIBLE) they show you a before image of a disheveled women with a team of professionals explaining what they are planning to do to change her hair, makeup and clothes, then at the end of the show while the team have been working so hard backstage they reveal the whole new transformation which always looks fantastic and takes ten years off their real age. Why is it that every time someone has a make over no matter how extreme they always love it? They never say "oh I don't like this colour", or "I hate the fringe" it just never happens. I would love to see someone appear with a shaved head.

I watched these make over's over and over again, I was mesmerized.

This is exactly what I wanted to do!!! I wanted the job of making somebody look and feel GREAT.

I wanted to be on TV doing all this myself.

But how the hell was I going to do it? Do I walk in to the TV studios? Or call them up on the phone for a nice chat? Bare in mind I was only sixteen/seventeen and I couldn't even cut hair yet let alone star on a UK television make over show. I must just say at this point that when we are at this age our minds can work in very mysterious ways and we always think that the unachievable is always achievable, which in hind sight actually is. So there, a little bit of useful information or not so useful depending on how you wish to look at it.

The only other problem with wanting to do this kind of work was that all the filming for this show was in London, after all, nothing exciting ever happened in Ripley.

No matter where I was or what I was doing all I could think about was breakfast TV. I was living the dream only I was living it out in my own imagination like a fantasy.

A few weeks later I was flicking through the back of a hair magazine in the classifieds where all the job applications could be found and one stood out more than any. It was an advert for an assistant to work for a front cover magazine styling the well known and rich 'n' famous for the photo shoots, so I immediately pulled out the page and set up my laptop to send an email of a possible job opportunity. It didn't matter if it was in London I'd deal with it if the time ever came, I'm sure I could work something out if I even stood a chance of receiving a reply. Again I had the rush and vibe like the first day of work, maybe because I saw it as a new project or that it was just another bee in the bonnet scenario but without any real thought I sent my e-mail with a click of a button and waited for a reply.

As usual the days went by at work and I was yet to receive a return mail when I checked my inbox every evening. I never told anyone about it although I was so desperate to tell someone about my hopeful adventure. I really wanted to keep the buzz I was feeling but I waited and waited and waited for a response.

There it was, sat in my inbox was the mail I had been waiting for. I was always quite a positive person so I was always hoping for the best in anything that I tried to do and this mail was no exception. I wouldn't say I was a competitive person but I wanted to do something with my life, something that gave me a satisfactory career move.

I quickly clicked on the mail and read the reply advising me to come and pay a visit to their offices in London for an interview. I was now in my element of excitement as I told my parents immediately. I think they were a little shocked at first, the thought that out of the blue I had just told them I had an interview in London but being the parents that they are they have never to this day doubted myself and are always prepared to support myself and my brother in the things that we do.

The day soon came round and there I was sat in the driving seat of my black ford fiesta with my dad heading down the M1 motorway towards London. It was a time when I had not long passed my driving test so I wanted to drive all the way. It was a long journey, longer than I had expected and there was me thinking I might have been able to get the bus myself. Half way on route to London unfortunately I got extremely bored holding on to the steering wheel and trying to keep my eyes open so my dad thankfully took over at the wheel and carried on the journey.

I was so happy that my dad was with me. It gave me a sense of security.

It seemed forever, no longer did the radio amuse me and the conversation with my dad had run dry. We'd already spoke about how I was getting on in my work place, life in general and what it would be like to be a millionaire was always a topic that I found intriguing and I became easily obsessed with and thinking about it, it was myself who would bring it up every time. We also spoke about how I thought things might be like when we arrived in London, if we ever got there, it was taking ages.

The M1 was just one long piece of concrete stretching for miles. It was long, boring and tiring just sitting watching streams of cars, lorries, tucks and vans speeding past wondering why they were all in such a rush to get where ever they were going.

When we finally reached London we found a car parking space just on the outskirts and travelled in using the subway. It actually seemed to get scarier, I was out of my comfort zone and in to new territory. I followed my dad closely not really knowing if my dad even knew were we were going which made me more nervous.

A thought turned to my dad. The thought about all this travelling to London with me, he was doing all this for me, he didn't have to drive me here he could have said no don't be stupid your not going but he didn't. He had taken a whole day off work just for me and as the thoughts were going through my mind it brought a slight lump to my throat.

The tube was busy in fact it was damn right hectic, people pushing and shoving arguing at not moving down the carriages. It was hot and sweaty. I thought why on earth if it gets this busy here in London don't they have this system more organized? It was something that later I was going to be asking myself over and over again in years to come.

We packed ourselves on to the tube train standing for what seemed like a lifetime, people were back to back, I was holding on to the rail but no one considered anyone. I knew if I let go of this hand rail I would never be able to reach it again. I held on to it tightly. No-one spoke to anyone just vacant eyes staring at one another or looking up in to mid air. A bead of sweat was running down the side of my cheek but I couldn't let go of the rail or move to wipe the heat from my forehead. Every one was more or less the same, the more you looked at someone sweating the hotter it made you feel. There were guys in suits sweating like mad and women perspiring trying to look as cool as cucumbers but again, the harder they tried the hotter it was becoming. Every stop that we reached more people tried to squeeze on but know one ever seemed to get off, every station was packed with people queuing to get on, it seemed almost impossible but people still found a space or gap to narrow themselves in to. This was a nightmare.

I knew if I let go of this hand rail I would get pushed further in to the carriage losing sight of my dad so I gripped as hard as I could until it was our turn to get off.

The doors eventually opened at our stop and we piled off, literally. Myself and my dad just stared at each other in relief of eventually getting off.

It was still busy, loud and racy on the platform, we headed to the escalators to make our way up to the street.

I'm sure escalators were designed for the simple reason for not having to walk up high stairs but people here were running up and down even though they didn't have too, it was crazy.

When we were above ground it was equally as busy but at least it was cooler than the carriages. There were people everywhere rushing around like some sort of important urgency, feet scattering over pavements, I couldn't quite get it in to my head that I was here in London. This world was big, much bigger than I was use too, I'd never been out of Ripley before so this was just something else, it made me think that this was a huge place and there was a much bigger world out there waiting for me. The buildings were huge towering blocks of concrete some with windows thirty to fifty floors high possibly more.

The traffic was horrendous too. Mini cabs or taxis as they are known in Derbyshire were everywhere almost like they had taken over from the luxury of having your own car this was enough to put any young kid off wanting to think about even learning to drive.

The noise of the traffic, people's feet rushing along the pavement and people talking on their mobile phones felt unusual, seeing things happening all at once was far too much to take in. Even the people looked weird, well, some of them anyway. It looked as if it didn't matter what you wore here there were so many people I guess doing their own thing that it wasn't important enough for them to care about what anyone else thought about each other, some of them had dressed so strangely it could have been possible that they hadn't even had time to look in the mirror before they had left home.

While we were walking the sights of people, buildings, sounds and scantiness of dodging out of the way of people seemed to take my mind off the whole point of being here. It made Ripley seem a tiny little home for me almost like just a scratch on the map. I bet people in London had never even heard of Ripley.

We walked for what seemed like miles cutting through streets going down narrow passages to cut through to yet more streets and crossing over parks where many people out of the near by offices seem to have lunch and take time out away from the stresses and strains of their paper work. As we carried on walking the busyness became less and less, we seemed to be walking away from the center of town and out in to a little more openness. Even though I hadn't a clue where I was going my dad thankfully did. He had done his research the night before and knew the ins and outs of which streets would lead to the streets we needed. As always, he was right! My feet were killing me yet my dad just powered on, I was tired yet I was younger than my dad obviously, surely it should have been the other way round.

Which brings me on to the subject of how come dads are always the last ones in the house to go to bed in the evenings? Normally mums go first, to get there beauty sleep of course and then the kids because you kept drifting off and your dad would tell you to go to bed and then your dad would be last, you see!

My dad used to stay up until the early hours of the morning watching TV, but when I used to catch him with his eyes closed I used to tell him to go to bed, but as always his answer back was that he wasn't asleep and was only resting his eyes. No matter what time in the early hours your parents would retire to bed they would always be up in the morning before yourself, even at weekends when you could have a lie in your parents never did, strange but true in most family life cases.

We arrived at a small mews lined with a cobbled surface, it was much quieter than the center as if know one knew about this rather quaint place. It was an enclosed area with a house at the end and an entrance door made of complete glass from top to bottom. As we approached the building the butterflies started to begin causing an unsettlement in my stomach as if they were out in force but I knew there was no going back, I'd brought my dad all this way and that was a big enough incentive for me to get to grips with the silvery chrome door handle, push hard and enter a completely new and different environment.

The reception was very different to the reception at work. It was on a much larger scale, more expensive looking and much more professional.

There was one male receptionist behind the desk and photos of front cover magazines plastered all over the wall behind him in glossy, reflective frames. I had never seen so many pictures, there were so many that you couldn't even tell the colour of the wall paper they were on. There were pictures of famous models, pictures of well known rock stars and even faces of royalty. I'd never been anywhere like this before. I felt that this time I was out of my element and took a step way too far out of my comfort zone. I shouldn't be here, this is all a mistake, these are serious people with serious jobs and then there's little old me, a nobody from a town know one had even heard of and classed as the north when really it was the midlands but I wasn't going to correct anyone's mistake in not knowing, after all, I felt I was nothing to these people. I nervously crept to the front of the reception, introduced myself and explained that I was here to see someone I had emailed. I was sweating profusely just trying to explain myself. I was winding myself up so much I made myself sound like I didn't know what I was talking about, after all I hadn't even spoke to this person before it was all done by a computer and a simple email. There was no getting out of this mess now.

We took a seat and waited until some one could see me. I have a vivid memory of being offered refreshments and my dad having a coffee so out of courtesy I had one too.

A short time later I was introduced to a woman in the correct field of interest I was concerned in and taken through corridors to an office, we all took a seat and the coffees were brought in by a smartly dressed assistant. I don't really know why on earth I said I'd have a coffee, not only was the underground boiling the walk to this place had about ruined me and now just the thought of drinking this damn coffee was melting me. Just looking at it made me sweat.

Dad on the other hand was as cool as a cucumber as ever, he sat there quiet and patiently while I explained the kind of things that I'd like to get involved in and also about what I had been doing since leaving school.

I don't know what came over me but I felt like the words were uncontrollably tumbling out of my mouth left, right and center.

I felt I had this very small period of time to get everything out of my mouth so I could impress her, I didn't want to loose this opportunity, I wanted to look positive and energetic, I wanted to prove I had it in me to succeed and now was the time to play my trump card.

I pulled out a small book with a few before and after picture of peoples hair that I had blow-dried which I thought might impress her but the thought of the pictures that were behind reception made me feel that my pictures where worthless but hey I gave it a go, I got the book out and continued to explain how and why I had done these so called hairstyles.

The women was very smartly dressed in a suit jacket and pencil skirt but she had a sternness and a slight arrogance about her, she only smiled when she found something amusing, one of those smiling or smirking moments for a better phrase was when I showed her my book of photographs.

I kind of saw it coming.

I felt the wetness of sweat under my shirt desperately trying not to look down just in case it was visible under my armpits.

As she flicked through my short book of pictures she explained in a round about way that she didn't take on anyone under the age of twenty five, I don't know how true that was but I think she had made her mind up the moment she laid her snake eyes on me in the reception, she went on and on about the staff she had working for her, how good and talented they all were and how detailed they saw creativeness in the work that they provided. Pretty much every thing that I said meant nothing to her, her time was her time and I was wasting it. I knew she was a busy women but I thought I'd of least be given a little credit for my efforts however by this point I wasn't just hot and sweaty I was dying of embarrassment, all my work that I thought was great she thought was less than average. I was gutted.

I was left with nothing to say apart from the usual thank you for taking the time to see me which you normally receive a reply of "it's a pleasure" but I didn't even get that, what did I expect after all, a job? I don't even think I finished my coffee but the meeting was clearly over and with a brisk wave of her finger pointed the way back to the reception to find our own way out.

One last look at the front covers and a nod to the receptionist and that was it, back out the way we came in. I know it wasn't an actual interview but all the things they taught me at school about going in to these kinds of situations, keeping calm and looking at them when they speak to you and listen when they are talking to you all went out the window as soon as I went in. All I could think about was how much of a sham and utter mess I must have made things look in there.

We stood outside a little to the left of the glass door in silence, I didn't know what to say or do.

I looked at my dad with an ocean of tears ready to explode out bulging beneath my eyes but I was trying so hard to hold them back that a lonely droplet fell on to my cheek. My dad comforted me as we walked out of the mews and back down the cobbled road. He was the opposite to me, so positive about how this was the first step and how much information she gave me on their kind of work they did, but I had nothing but negative issues with what had just taken place. I guess it's easy to blame others when their not around you but I was so two faced about her when I got out of the building yet I did my best to be polite to her while I was in the same room. I've learnt, since that situation in life, you don't always get what you want, although, if you try hard enough there are always ways to get to there.

Walking around London discussing the situation and babbling on about life in general we stopped for some lunch in a pub. It was a traditional London pub so my dad said, with the layout of the pub and the design of the bar it had hardly been redesigned in to one of these modern, trendy bars you get today, it also had a door that read 'smoking room' well, I wished I hadn't of asked because another thing with dads is that once you ask them about something you always get the whole history of how things all began and what people back in the day used things for, how it was used and all that boring stuff as a kid you don't really care about and the so called smoking room was no exception, at the end of the day this was all before my time but still he went on and on, the least I could do was listen and look interested for if it wasn't for him I wouldn't be here sat in the pub in Gloucester Road in the first place.

To say we hadn't eaten since breakfast I wasn't all that hungry, maybe because I was left with a sickly feeling inside when I left the room earlier, however I managed to stuff down a ploughman's lunch which arrived in a tireless effort from the kitchen as if we was a little to late for lunch and the chef had gone home so they scrambled together what ever they could find to try and make a meal somewhat edible, especially for the eight pound fifty price tag that came with it. I don't want to sound ungrateful but after that remark it probably sounds like I am.

Why is it every thing you buy here in London is

so damn expensive, I mean the coffee we had when we arrived was three quid and who on earth has a 'croissant' for breakfast, southerners ha! I mean what ever happened to the good old fashioned bacon and egg butty eh? And back in the day back to ye olde bread and dripping yuk!!! It was an olden day thing however I think old people still do this kind of thing today, their the ones who kept telling you when you were younger "it'll put hairs on your chest", but to this day I have never believed that remark. After all, there has been no women under the age of at least thirty that I have ever come across having hairs on her chest let alone had they ever sat there eating dripping.

After lunch we took a stroll around the London sights not only to walk off our heavy lunch of blocks of cheese and tidy chunks of bread but there was nothing left for us to do, it was like we came we saw and now nothing, we didn't even conquer. It was like there had become an emptiness. All the preparation, the long drive on the endless concrete road, the never ending walk to get here and now that was it, for what? Absolutely nothing.

I must admit it couldn't of been all that bad, the sights were great I'd never been here before so seeing Big Ben and Westminster was outstanding. The boats on the River Thames and the amount of pigeons in Trafalgar square was fascinating, I felt like I knew and understood these surroundings, after all I had seen them before but only in the film Mary Poppins, the only thing was I didn't feed the birds like they did because the bird seed was about a quid, scrounging gets, people will sell anything here, even bloody bird seed.

Today, unfortunately the birds have now been scared away from Trafalgar Square and no more bird seed is sold to tourist due to the birds making such a mess. In hindsight I can now see the moral behind this but don't worry for those bird lovers out there, there are still many pigeons in other parts of London. As a tip though, bring your own seed.

After a while we wandered down Park Lane, my feet were tired and I was becoming more and more lethargic however it was somewhere my dad wanted to go to look at the car garages along the busy road. It seemed a lot less hectic on the pavements here however the never ending constant flowing of traffic was continuous. He explained how this street was well known for its glitzy hotels and famous guests that stayed in them and that it was one of the most expensive areas in London to live. I only understood because of the number of times I had played the board game Monopoly, as when you brought Park Lane you already felt you had won the game even if you ended up being the old boot, I just thought it was all expensive around here.

We walked down Park Lane stopping at every car dealership on the street, I didn't know how anyone could become so indulged in looking at cars, I mean he wasn't going to buy one at 100,000 a pop, its just not normal. I was seventeen at the time remember and a lot has changed with me since then, cars do play a slight priority in my life now. How things change.

I moaned dis-heartedly as we paused yet again to see another piece of metal on wheels, I knew nothing about cars neither was it something on my list to do in London. I had lost interest and all I wanted to do was sit down and take my shoes off which surprisingly did still have some rubber on their soles after the trek we had walked.

As we got half way down Park Lane we reached a petrol station where my dad made the decision to take a detour and go down a street on the right hand side. I asked where we were going now but it clearly looked as though he also had lost his bearings and he too was in his own mind saying to himself that he didn't know either. We carried on walking past Purdeys gun store and other shops I had never heard however once again dads have this kind of auto pilot brain in telling you how high profile the names above the doors of the shop fronts actually are. It was like an old school education lesson in history and I hated history.

We reached the bottom of the street and I had almost given up on walking any further when before my very eyes in such luck and I mean utter coincidence there it was, the salon I had been seeing on the TV Programs where they did all the morning makeovers. I couldn't believe it. I was pulled towards the window of the red bricked salon like a magnet a canopy shading the sun over my head. I looked through the window with such anticipation forgetting how close the window was to my fore head and bumping my head trying hard to make it look like nothing had happened to save myself from any further embarrassment.

Leaning over the vibrant flower boxes resting proudly on the window sill I starred inside with amazement. There was a busyness inside of what I presumed was a mixture of stylists and juniors scurrying around, some shampooing at the backwashes at the far end of the salon and some just standing next to stylists, hang on a minute, the stylist were sitting down on stools attached to wheels while they were cutting hair, now this was something I'd never seen before. In my hairdressers we got told off if we sat down but here it just seemed pretty natural.

My dad stood next to me peering through glancing at the activity in front of us, it was almost like watching a show only this one we didn't have to pay for.

I was so intrigued in what I was seeing I could barley take my eyes away trying desperately hard not to steam up the window with breathing my own carbon dioxide on to it so I slowly prized myself away, but I only managed to creep closer towards the front of the salon towards the door for a casual glance in at the reception. I walked slower than slow to try and take in every moment that I had. I didn't want this chance to pass although it seemed to pass sooner than I would have liked. It wasn't as though I could just stand there gleaming in like a lost boy looking for someone to take me in but my brain was telling me to go further.

It was going to be the biggest and scariest decision I was going to make.

We crossed over the road to the park where we sat for a while in the midday sun.

The park seemed somewhat quiet, it seemed to be a million miles away from the outside world. I couldn't get my head around that from the levels of traffic in this concrete city the park seemed to be a relaxed green heaven environment yet was only a stones throw from the road around it, almost like an island with a running track all the way around it only it was the rush of traffic in the race.

The park was called Berkley Square also famous for a song that was once wrote called A Nightingale Sang In Berkley Square, a song my dad once brought for me on sheet music and pestered me to play it time and time again on the piano. I never did learn that piece of music and I am also ashamed to say neither do I know how it goes.

I will get to know it one day.

I bombarded my dad with questions about the salon expecting him to some how know the answers.

What he thought it would be like working there? How many people he thought worked there? Did he think the man himself worked there? Did he think the man himself was there now? The list went on and on and on, unfortunately the answers came a little less quickly than the questions.

When I refer to the man himself I'm talking about the owner of the salon, he was the one on TV doing the make over shows, he cuts the hair of the rich and famous he was the most successful stylist in the UK and beyond, in my eyes he was the ultimate hairdresser.

My dad sat there talking to me while soaking up the sun and also taking five minutes to rest his feet. Although he kept talking I must be honest I wasn't really listening as the cogs in my brain were working hard to think about my next move.

"That's it!!!!" I need to go in, another one of my useless off the wall ideas but the only way to see more of the salon was to actually get inside. My dad was less excited about the idea which was a little understandable, it was like the scene from Billy Elliot when the young boy tells his dad he really wants to become a ballet dancer as he enters the audition room and the look on his dads face tells a story as if to say "and what on earth are you going to do once your in there"?

I hadn't thought of that but I'm sure something would crop up once in the moment.

We sat for about half an hour and debated making a move to start heading back home to the midlands but by this point I still hadn't made my mind up and I also wasn't ready to leave the salon in the distant background, I just wasn't ready to turn my back on the salon I had dreamt of one day being able to work in.

I couldn't just say to myself go in but neither could I make a decision on getting up and leaving.

I stood up, looked at my dad and told him I was going to ask if I could take a look around the salon and for him to wait in the park. I don't know what possessed me to do this alone after my dad had been at my side whenever I went to do anything before, but with a heavy, stubborn foot I walked out of the dusty, gravel stoned park up the steps and on to the pavement ready to cross back over the road to the salon.

I stood waiting for the traffic to clear but it seemed endless, I must have been waiting for what felt like at least ten minutes but there was no gap in the traffic which left me with nothing to do but wait. I changed my mind several times whilst waiting, I felt like I had an angel on one side of me telling me to go on I'll be fine and a devil on the other saying what a bad idea this was and I'll be turned down before I even reach the reception and with a puff of cartoon smoke you see in the movies both angel and devil had disappeared out of my head and off of my shoulders.

Within time there was a short pause and I crossed the road nearing ever closer to the red brick building on the corner of the square. It was only a few yards in front of me when I could see the glass windows reflecting an overall expensiveness out on to the street. The dazzling displays of products on the window shelves taking pride of place encouraging members of the public on the outside world to indulge them in to buying the best products in the hair care world. The sign above the door was ornate with class, it was a wooden sign with gold writing and the logo slightly swinging in the breeze catching your attention to detail of where I was about to walk beneath.

I walked passed a couple of times and glanced

in once again through the window, it was still as busy and energetic as before. It was then I realized that it was now or never and there was no chance I was going to back down now. I had been treated badly at my salon by a few of the staff and let down with so called friends, but the excitement of coming to London started to lift my spirit, I was also gutted about my original meeting   but fortunately all this negativity gave me a huge kick up the backside, the thought of being turned down, but to top it all off I had just walked passed my dream job at the salon I really wanted work in. I was here. it was now or never, and then with one small step for mankind and one giant deep breath by the young boy that I was, I found a split second gasp of confidence as I stepped in to a whole new experience and a whole new level of hair salon and hairdressing.

I walked calmly in to the reception. It was a rounded wooden reception desk with a marble top like something you would expect to see on the Titanic.

There were three receptionists, all female with make up done to perfection and smiles you only usually see when you buy them something nice like a new handbag or pair of shoes.

I smiled back and I was asked if they could help me.

"Yes hi, I'm James and I've come to see the owner"

"Ok James is it for a hair cut today?"

"Errrmmmm no, its for a meeting"

At this point I had already put my foot in things,

why couldn't I just come out with the comment I'm here regarding any junior jobs? That would have been easy or could I have an application form please? Now that would have been even easier, but no, I chose the difficult route which only lead to more questions for me to answer.

She pulled out a clip board with a piece of headed paper displaying the salon branded logo at the top with a list of names upon, I knew I wasn't a name that was on the list but I just stood there as if my name was going to be read out like in school.

"James" she said, does he know you're here today"?

And with that I replied "yes". What was I thinking?

I could see her looking up and down the clip board searching for my name but to no avail as I stood in front of her like a lost soul.

I was told to take a seat while she went upstairs to find out.

I sat down on a huge leather sofa, so huge that my feet didn't touch the floor. I looked up and in front of me was a spiral staircase leading to another floor. Pictures hung from top to bottom of the salon in gold and gilt picture frames and music was blasting from the speakers above. People were working on the ground floor and a few staggering looks came my way as if to say who are you seeing today which I was asked a couple of times by the juniors, I had to explain I was waiting for the receptionist.

A chandelier draped over the stair case and an element of class and wealth shone through the glistening glass droplets coming from the ceiling above or could they be real crystals? Nothing was to surprise me here.

I waited absorbing the atmosphere worrying about what I had got myself in to, waiting for what the outcome was going to be, would I be asked to leave? I just didn't know. The sweaty palms and beady forehead started to appear and it wasn't long before I had to take off my coat in a fashionable manner trying to look as if I was meant to be here.

Clients and staff were walking around constantly, they were coming from all directions, some from upstairs some off the ground floor and some were coming up from a downstairs basement, there must have been another floor beneath me. This was the biggest salon I had ever stepped foot in before.

I watched as clients came to reception to pay their bills with their newly coiffured hair. The hair cuts weren't just the normal hair cuts but actual styles I'd never seen walk out of a salon before, they were certainly without a doubt far better than the cuts we could produce at the local salon back home in Derbyshire.

Another thing I noticed was almost every client paying their bill were also buying products by the dozen, this was something else we struggled to do in our salon. I always thought selling a product was like pushing a deal, trying to get a client to buy something that they really didn't want and could get cheaper from the pound shop but here it was the opposite, there was no hard sell. They seemed to buy whatever they needed and at any cost. I guess I too would have brought anything just to get a carrier bag with the logo and name on it just to say I'd been there too.

I kept looking up at the stair case waiting for the receptionist to come back down. It was taking a while and I was becoming more irritable with the sweat running down my neck patiently trying to keep calm whatever the out come.

The receptionist came back down the stair case happily gliding down as if she'd done it a million times before.

"James darling, can I ask what it is regarding"?

"I'm looking for a job as a junior" I replied.

That was it!!! That is all I was meant to say in the beginning.

I said how I had travelled all the way from Derbyshire to come here which I know was a lie but hey, it was only a little white one so it didn't count but I'm sure she had never heard of the place especially as she wasn't English herself. She did say she would let the boss know and it would be something it would be sure to impress him. I smiled with a smile from cheek to cheek, I also believed her.

She gave me a piece of paper and a pen to write my details on and explained they would be in touch.

I scribbled away trying to write in my best handwriting to make it as readable as possible, I didn't want them not to be able to read my details, I was so desperate to put as much information down about myself so that there was no way they couldn't reach me.

I handed the receptionist the paper, showed my appreciation and said my Thankyou's.

'We'll be in touch' she replied.

I walked out with a brave smile on my face and rushed over the road carefully not to get run over and entered the park where my dad was doing his old trick of pretending not to be asleep. I couldn't wait to explain to him what I had done.

He seemed really happy for me and also relieved that I was back in one piece and after filling him in we started walking back to the station to find where we had parked the car for the long journey home.

On the way home we chattered most of the way excitable at what I had achieved today. I couldn't believe I had stood for about twenty minutes or more in the grandest salon in Mayfair. I felt more relieved that I hadn't wasted my dad's time as well because he had taken the time out of his own work commitments for me to come to London in the first place. I know my dad wouldn't be disappointed in any way regardless to the out come whether it was a pointless journey or not. My mum and dad have never made myself or my brother feel like anything that we have done in life has been pointless, mistakes that we've made and times we didn't listen have never been frowned upon, they have just been the way parents should be in supporting their children in all the activities that they choose to do. Normal parents.

The rest of the journey I was asleep probably releasing the energy from my excited mind. It had been a tiring day for us both and getting home and in to bed ready to go back to work tomorrow was something I wasn't looking forward too.

I couldn't wait to tell my mum all about my London adventure, but by the time we arrived home it was late and she had already turned the lights off and headed to bed so I knew it would have to wait until the morning.

I went straight to bed thinking about my adventurous day in London.

The next day I awoke in the glee of telling all to my mum but unfortunately she had already left for work so yet again my story had to wait.

I set off for work, it was cold and wet the rain was a drizzling mist which added more to the dreamy thought of being in such a comfortable bed. My mind was still on being in London. I walked along the pavement thinking to myself that I have yet to pass anyone on the street neither was there a rushing of feet, no busy roads and no bleeping horns, it was so different to London life there was no edge or motivation for going to work today, thinking about it the only thing that Ripley had that London didn't was singing birds, there wasn't even any in Berkley Square but we had them in Crosley park.

I never said anything at work about my day off, no one asked and so I didn't let on. All day I was comparing the things that we did at our salon to the one in London, everything seemed so backward and less organized. Looking around no one really had anything in common with each other and no one was really any ones true genuine friend. I didn't really spot it before but now I had seen a different side to hairdressing it stuck out like a sore thumb.

The day however was much like any other, I took a lot of stick from the juniors and was pushed out of conversations as per usual as the juniors talked about staff behind others backs. It became second nature to be treated in this way but I knew I had to just grin and bare it.

This salon was small in comparison, less glitzy and not at all glamorous. The only thing to leave this salon in an almost glamorous way was Mrs. Smith with her usual perm and Sheila with her brushed out, back combed set with half a ton of hairspray to provide extra hold, and we thought that was how to style hair.

It was the same people day in day out and the same conversations constantly. I wanted this salon to be like the one in London but I knew it was never going to live up to that standard.

I thought I'd try my hand at selling a product, I saw them doing it in London so why couldn't I do that here? I told myself that the next shampoo I did I would talk about the client's hair and scalp, what kind of products they used at home? And did they need any to take home with them today? I thought I'd skip the holiday and the weather bit for once.

Well once I sold my first product they just kept on buying, it was as if they had been needing someone to advise them on what they should be using and how they should be using products at home, I felt maybe for the first time they were having a completely different conversation to the normal rehearsed shampoo conversation routine, they felt for once that someone actually cared about their hair in a different way. They seemed to like it.

Unfortunately it was short lived as along with success came jealousy and it didn't help me in the junior department as they were aware I was doing something different, something that wasn't positive to them. I soon stopped trying hard at what I did. It was a shame because I actually cared about what I did but no-one saw what was going on behind the scenes.

Every night I finished work I'd run home to see if I had any post via London but every night to no avail. It was frustrating and maybe just maybe I might even be doing a career that wasn't meant for me. I had always been told that if you fall down twice you were to get up a third time and it was that little saying that kept me in the game of hairdressing. I felt like I was being knocked down several times a day.

I taught myself that failing was easy, anyone can fail but success was hard and didn't come easily to many, but I didn't want easy, I always did things the hard way.

Days went by with nothing in the mail.

One day as I was at work on my knee's wiping the skirting boards with a damp worn out cloth marking the walls leaving a faint dirt mark behind from the rag, I felt a buzzing in my pocket. It was my mobile phone, I wasn't really meant to have it on me whilst in working hours but I always had it in my pocket on vibrate and silent rather than a ring tone so that know one would hear.

I quickly and quietly hurried and hid myself in the bathrooms, it was my mum. She never used to call me on my mobile whilst I was at work but I thought what the hell and answered the phone.

"You've got a letter" she said

"Really, who's it from"?

"How the bloody hell do I know I haven't opened it"?

"Oh".

"It says it's from London" she said.

"Open it, open it" I calmly whispered as I was still supposed to be out in the corridor cleaning.

I could hear her rustling the envelope as she tried to open it,

"read it then, what does it say"?

There seemed to be a moment of hesitation as she paused making me more nervous and then she said,

"They want you to go to work there for a week's trial next week"

"You're joking"? I couldn't believe my luck I thought they had forgotten about me or wasn't interested but here I am in the toilet next to the blue bottle of thick bleach talking with my mum sharing a moment of joy who'd of believed it?!!!

I hung up the phone put it back in my pocket and carried on with my cleaning, it all started to seem so worth while putting up with the shit just to hear some positive news.

I knew that receptionist would pass on my message I just knew it.

Opening the door as I got home there it was the letter I was waiting for right in front of me on the table.

I read it over and over again just to make sure that I was reading it correctly, now all I had to do was to tell my boss that I needed next week off and unfortunately the only way I could do it was to tell her the truth and I couldn't wait.

Wednesday came and I plucked up the courage to ask the manageress if I could have a word with her after work. It took me a while to approach her because every time I went to talk to her she was either bufonting someone's hair in to some kind of unusual yet creative sculpture or talking to members of staff. In any case it always seems that walls have ears and soon the word had already began to murmur around the salon about our little meeting when a junior asked me what I was having a meeting for after hours, maybe she was worried I was going to grass one of them up and only now did they start to panic. Of course I never did tell her why.

I sat in the salon and explained the situation to her. She looked pleasantly surprised but also intrigued about what I had done, her eyes staring everywhere but at mine. I could tell she was looking to ask questions but I quickly hurried her on her decision to give me the time off, after all it wasn't as if I was leaving to work elsewhere I was merely going for another work experience week and she was left with no option than to agree as long as I came back and told them all about it afterwards. Little did I know the consequences.

I was sat in the hotel room in London's South Kensington that my dad had organized for me. It was very plush with my own shower room and breakfast facilities. We walked a practice walk to the salon the day before as I knew tomorrow when my dad had left I was going it alone and needed to know which route I was heading for.

It was all so new and nerve racking to me that I had a fall out with my dad early in the morning due to me not wanting to use a tube or a bus to get there because I didn't know what to do and where to get off etc....

The only other way was to walk an hour's walk and in hindsight I should have just listened to what I was told and used transport.

It took a lot longer to walk than I had expected although in the sun it did seem a nice walk passing through some of the sights I had seen the last time I visited. We went through Hyde Park and past the Royal Albert Hall over a river and through the park on to Park Lane. It was when I got to Park Lane I had remembered the way from before, past the car garages up to the petrol station and turn right. I was talking my way through the directions in my head as we walked on just to be sure I could remember the way on my own.

Looking back it was such a long way to walk but I guess not listening to my dad was a typical common occurrence I had, a father and son thing.

Once back at the hotel I said my goodbyes to my dad and he left. It felt strange seeing the back of the car leaving me in the distance until he reached the end of the road and turned left, he was gone, the sight of the last remaining number of his number plate bringing a small lump to the back of my throat and a swelling of tears glistening in my eyes.

I sat in my room on my own. It was quiet apart from the constant drone of traffic outside. It had also become suddenly lonely, part of me was sad and another happy about my first day tomorrow but all I could think about was home, which was strange after I had barley just arrived.

I remember lying on the bed thinking time was passing so slowly, I made myself a cup of coffee from the simple yet trusted complementary on the bed side table and decided to call my mum to let her know my dad was on his way back. We chattered about what we did that day and to make sure I'd be careful, all the kind of things your mum's worry about, and with that the conversation was running dry. She wished me luck and we said our goodbyes, I told her I would call her tomorrow once I got back to the hotel.

I woke up early on Monday morning, put on my new trousers and tucked in my shirt after using all the condiments and miniatures in the bathroom. I groomed my hair spending a little bit more time than I usually would, after all I wanted to make a good impression on my first day. I think I must have checked myself in the mirror several times before I left the hotel room, a little O.C.D maybe but it made me feel better.

The nerves as always where there too, but this

was something I really wanted to do and so with my head held high and a little too much aftershave I left the building and started my long journey to the salon.

I arrived at the salon extremely early, the walk was brisk and the weather was dry but fresh. I was cheerful at the thought of going to work at one of the most well known salons in London. I passed all the places I had walked by the day before with my dad, turned left at the petrol station and on to the street of the salon.

I was both nervous and excited when walking being careful not to trip and scuff my new shoes whilst being nosey looking through all the windows of the expensive shops.

Once I arrived I pushed open the heavy wooden door and entered the salon where I was met by the floor manager, I couldn't actually believe I was standing here, I was in the salon and I was going to be here for the next five days.

I was shown around the salon by the manager, it was magical to see each floor and also the bits that the clients never saw, I was introduced to some of the other juniors and I was told to shadow one of them during the day. It seemed that the juniors had to be in the salon earlier than the stylists, this was so the salon could be set up professionally before the stylists or clients arrived. To me it already looked professional as not one piece of it was out of place but once the silver plated tissue boxes, products and equipment was set out the salon looked different altogether.

I was briefly shown the ropes and told not to hold back if things needed doing, what they meant was don't wait to be asked. Already I knew I was good at that.

I tried so desperately hard to remember everything I was told as there was so much to take in.

The first clients steadily proceeded to come through the reception doors as it turned 9am and the stylists were up at their sections and in position ready to take control of their day. Every stylist had their own section, own mirror and own brushes where in our salon we had to share most things and sit in whatever section's were free but these guys made the whole service from consultations to showing them the back of their hair with a mirror absolutely tailor made, even down to the art of juniors delicately shampooing the clients with the correct shampoo and conditioner's and spending the whole of their time and attention on the clients instead of themselves.

What I'd of done to sit in a stylists chair and have my hair cut in a silky, shiny, clean smelling gown. Arhhh, bliss I thought.

That day I did similar things that I was used to like sweeping up hair after a hair cut had finished but even that was done with more skill and drive almost as if synchronized.

Coffee, tea, breakfast and lunch was constantly being brought out to clients on silver trays by the salon caterers. Everything about this salon was like pure gold, like being Royalty for the day. The music was on and the dryers were just as loud but the constant chatter about hair, colour and ideas brought a new concept to the conversations rather than what I was used to like talking about the weather and holidays.

The stylists were so much more superior than I'd ever seen, so much more in to their work, just watching them you could clearly see they enjoyed what they did. To them it wasn't like work it was more like a hobby which was exactly how I saw it every time I got up in the morning.

Everyone during the day at some point asked me about my interests, I felt part of a team for once and it was only my first day, it felt right, it felt like I was meant to be here all along and that every time I was told to take a break I didn't want to, I didn't want to miss a trick, I just wanted to be stood on the floor every minute of the day learning the skills from the sculptured hairdressers before me, food was the last thing on my mind. I was so pleased I missed my lunch break as for what was about to come was the entire highlight of my day.

There was a salon activeness, a different junior racing around the salon cleaning and preparing equipment like no other. Brushes were being laid out on a towel and products set out in complete preciseness, tongs, rollers and hairdryers placed on sections with accuracy. It all seemed very professional for the climax I'd been waiting for. It was like experiencing Disney land for the very first time only I was seventeen.

Water prays were filled and placed on the sections along with magazines and a drink before a client was seated in the chair and treated like the queen.

The assistant waited at the side of this client arms held behind his back patiently waiting for a stylist to appear. And then, from a swung open door speedily walking over to this client was the man himself, the celebrity hairstylist I was long awaiting to see. He glided across the salon as if on ice or even air. His long hair, glamorous clothing all adding to the luxury of having him cut and style your hair. Straight away he looked like he knew exactly what he was doing, he stood out among the other stylists the elegance of the way he moved and worked was unbelievably mesmerizing. I couldn't believe I was stood in his salon watching him working his magic delicately running his hands through the client's hair paying high attention to her every need. This had been something I had only ever seen on the TV before and now here I was intensively watching it for real. The goose bumps on my arms, hair stood on its end I felt like I was part of something incredible.

His flair and aura was magical, however there seemed to be a vague distance between the connection of himself and his clients. He swished his hair whilst explaining theirs in the consultation and spoke a lot using his hands to explain what he had in mind. His consultation seemed detailed all the way down to sketching out of his ideas on paper which gave the client an accurate account of his thoughts. The client seemed to sit in complete satisfaction even though he hadn't even started the hair cut itself, she too could see a magical outline of the performance that was going to be taking place and with that she was led to the backwash by the assistant to have her hair therapeutically washed.

Once the client was washed and seated back in the chair I watched as he sat on the cutting stool sectioning the hair and cutting with great accuracy. His flowing hands holding each section whipping the hair up in to the air and cutting effortlessly.

He spoke continuously whilst cutting so much so that the client seldom had to speak but I don't think the client would have minded, she too was watching at the hair changing form and taking its new shape, it was as therapeutic as day dreaming and in no time the cut was dried off and ready for styling. I couldn't believe that these women were like putty in his hands

Products and electricals were passed over like a surgeon asking for his tools, everything was placed in a clean and tidy manner. The hair was dressed out and the final spray was added finishing the look that he had sketched out previously on paper which I must say was spot on and very accurate.

The client didn't even have to say a word, the smile and the glisten in her eyes was enough to say she had never felt an experience like it. She was happy the stylist was happy and above all I was over the moon.

I watched as he did client after client not stopping for a break just continuously snipping away from one client to another, I was in my element, I just loved to see this guy cutting and styling in such a charismatic way. It was like he could dance with the hair and communicate with the client telepathically.

This kept a permanent smile on my face through out the rest of the day.

I wish I could speak to him or touch his scissors I know I was being a little too absorbed but I couldn't get it in to my thick scull that I was seeing all of this for real.

That day I was in the back room. The back room was a room away from the clients where all the used towels, trays with refreshments on and rubbish was discarded and also where you could slip away if you needed a little time out or sit down.

I was stood in the back when the door flung open and in front of me stood the man himself, this was the celebrity stylist to the stars, he spoke with a soft and gentle voice sniffing as if he had a cold or a runny nose and then he asked me who I was and how I was getting on to which I answered with a nervous persona. We shook hands as he welcomed me to his salon not really paying attention to me as his eyes focused on everything but me and back out he went on to the salon floor to continue his clients.

I didn't mind the fact that he didn't really look at me as I was just so ecstatic that he saw me and I actually got to meet him, however it would have been nice to have got an autograph but I didn't want to push my luck.

I stood in amazement, it was the first time I had been up close and personal with a celebrity before, my mind rewinding the conversation in my head over and over again even if it was a brief encounter, I had just met my idle and I was the happiest boy in town. All I wanted to do was jump up and down and tell every one in the salon I had just spoke to him but I managed to keep it under raps thinking to myself that these people see him every day and didn't seem to have the same reaction that I did when I met him. It seemed that to everyone in the salon he was just a normal guy like the rest of them doing clients back to back and providing a service so I thought it must have been that first time moment of meeting him and it would soon wear off, but it never really did.

I had idolized this stylist for such a long time and I was in a place where I longed to be forever.

It was really quiet sad but I didn't want this day to end.

The day flew by and before long I was back in my hotel room lying on the bed exhausted, not only had I been on my feet all day but I had been awake since 6am and I had walked half way across London twice, but not exhausted enough to call my parents and tell them what I had seen and done during the day.

I had a little to eat and went straight to bed setting my alarm as not to forget to get up the next day for another day at the office as they say.

The week was one of the quickest weeks I had ever worked, I enjoyed every moment watching and learning and seeing my celebrity stylist pampering his clientele.

Towards the end of the week I was getting stylist telling me how efficient and helpful I was, the juniors found themselves attached to me as I did them. I felt wanted and liked for once, I really felt that this time I was part of one big family, part of the team.

We worked all day, trained in the evening and socialized with a few drinks after work. this seemed to be a regular occurrence.

There was no jealousy between any of the staff which I never really understood with there being around sixty people working together under one roof.

In my salon at home there was about ten of us and some days you could cut the atmosphere with a knife. People thought they where higher than others or better than others only it was a shame the manager never saw what was going on behind the scenes but here everyone was on the same level, everyone was friends with each other and everyone above all got on. Everyone worked together sharing their ideas and helping each other out, they all seemed to care. No matter how many different characters there seemed to be, there was no bad tensions or animosity.

Finally the week came to an end and it was time to pack my things and go home.

My parents came to the salon to pick me up. They waited outside in the park opposite where myself and my dad originally had sat when I contemplated walking in to the Mayfair salon in the beginning. I had waited in the salon as long as I could that evening locking every memory I had in to my mind in case I was never to return again.

I wanted to remember everything from the working day to the décor. I absorbed as much as possible taking one last look around whilst walking slowly down the staircase sliding my hand down the golden arm of the brass hand rail in the hope that I didn't have to wash this hand ever again.

I said my good-byes to the manager and also to whoever was left in the salon and I reached out one last time to the lion headed door knob to head back to my parents in the park.

I felt both happy and sad that I had completed my week but now I had to go home.

I was shattered, my legs felt stiff my feet ached and my overall body was tired yet strangely it was the best I had felt in a long while.

We drove home that evening talking almost all the way about my week in the salon. Once again my parents were proud of me and I knew there was going to be a lot of questions to come but for now all I wanted to do was get home and in to bed knowing I had a rest day on Sunday, although normal work resumed on Monday as usual at the salon I hated. I know the word hate is a very strong word but that was the only word to describe the way I felt about that place at the time.

Work at my salon commenced at 8.30am and I knew as soon as I arrived there was going to be questions that needed answers. I could tell that every one already knew about my week and where I had been because as the staff started filtering through the salon they looked at me in surprise and

71

spoke to me as if I was their long lost friend, almost as if they wanted to be my best friend intrigued to know about how I had got on and what it was like.

All day I had stylists moseying around me whenever they got chance to a free moment hanging in on anything that came out of my mouth but I kept things simple not to let on too much, some what cagey so not to share too much of what was my experience. It was kind of selfish of me in a way but I didn't care. It was me who did my homework and it was me who made the step to travelling all the way to London, not them. They could have done the same but unfortunately with working with them every day it wasn't hard to see that none of them had the nerve to not only leave Ripley for new prospects but not even for only a day. It was like they were happy and quaint in doing the same old thing day in day out, but for me it was boring, I needed that extra excitement of seeing glitz and glamour I just wanted to shout out "there's so much more to hairdressing but you guys will never find out if you don't get out there"!!! But hey, that was my opinion and I kept it to myself. The staff in this salon were very narrow minded and could only see so far.

During the working day I tried to keep myself to myself as the juniors had got slightly pissed of with the attention I was gaining in the morning with the stylists. Time went slow not only was I clock watching but I found it dull. I couldn't even wait to take an hour's lunch break just to get out of the salon, one thing that didn't ever occur to me when I was in the London salon.

Things were different for me from this day forward as all I kept doing was comparing the two salons.

I was sad at work which created a change in attitude at home. All I wanted to do was quit yet the thought of packing up and leaving to go to London was out of the question, it was a scary thought I mean, how would I afford to live? Where would I live? It was a huge place and I had no friends or family there.

When you're younger and living at home you never have to think about moving away from your parents, you can never actually believe that you will ever be without them. You think they will be by your side, paying your bills and doing you're washing forever, so thinking about going to London was not on the menu for me, it wasn't even a possibility. So I thought.

I worked as normal until 6pm Friday. I met with a friend in my local for a quick drink before I went home for a super fast tea, wash and change before I then met up again with my mates for a typical Friday night out on the town.

By the way a typical night out for me as a seventeen year old would be very much 'the norm' for the majority of this age group, which is drink as much as possible with as little money as possible and keep up with your mates. Also pretend you enjoy drinking beer, order a takeaway on the way home and throw it all back up,,,,,,, GREAT!!!!!! And you know what? We've all been there and said we would never do it again.

However, this night it wasn't to be as I was head straight constantly thinking about my career.

When I got home leaning up on the bread bin was a gold coloured envelope, the same envelope I had received before from London with my name across the front. It was sealed along with the logo and emblem of the London salon running across the top of the seal.

I opened it quickly but carefully trying hard not to tear the emblem as it meant so much to me. I pulled out the piece of A4 paper and opened it.

My eyes lit up with delight, while I read down the paper my mum and dad asking me what it said.

I knew what it said, I knew exactly what it said but I read it again out loud for them to hear it.

It was a congratulations letter saying that I had earned myself a full time job in London at the salon I dreamt to work in all my life, my work ethic and determination during that week had impressed them. It was once again a proud moment for us all to share as a family, and with a start date on the letter alot of thought needed to be taken in to account in a very short space of time as to what was the right decision to make.

I read the letter over and over again my mind partly ecstatic another confused, it took a lot out of me believing that this was all so very true.

The weeks went by but I said nothing to the people at my current salon with my mum and dad still waiting on a decision from me. Nothing was said in or outside of work.

I thought about it every day, to be honest there

wasn't a moment when I didn't think about it.

I asked myself why would I move from Derbyshire to London? What would be the advantages and disadvantages? yet I guess I was much more bias at the thought of staying put. I really wanted to work there but I also wanted to be around my family and friends. I loved being around people I knew and my social life was excellent here.

In time through many conversations I asked my mates what they thought they would do if they were in the same position to which most of their answers being go and do it, there was never a question about it with them, it just seemed as though they just wanted to move on to the next pub for another beer and talk about the usual topics of sport, women, cars, women, sport and so on. I also asked the family and they too said it would be a golden opportunity. I don't know what my problem was, I knew in my heart I wanted to do it but there was a little part of me saying to myself that If I had the slightest of doubts don't go, but I wanted to. There was just no pleasing me.

After a night out on the town with my friends I ended the night with a typical Ripley kebab and a slow stroll home with one of my mates talking about our futures. We discussed where we'd like to be in ten years time wishing our lives away before our time, ageing ourselves with every step. When us guys seem to have alot to drink we do seem to talk about the most spaced out, weird things, it doesn't matter what any of our opinions are as the next morning we have usually forgotten about all the gibberish stories we told, it's just the way we are, it kind of comes with the male territory I guess, and also when all you've done is drank all night you seem to get the munchies where by you can eat almost anything so the kebab went down a treat. Word of advice,,,,, never eat one sober.

Eventually the conversation turned to myself, London and the salon.

We got to the end of the road and talked for a while, I suppose we were talking loudly instead of what we thought was quietly with it being the early hours knowing that we had been underage drinking, but one thing was said that helped make me seem to either sober up or knock some sense in to me, something that all of a sudden I related to drunk or not.

He said "James, given the opportunity you would be stupid not to go, even if you don't like it at least you've tried it, know one else has the balls to go and do it."

I don't know what it was but it made me think about what I really wanted, it made me feel like it was time to get serious and grow up a little. It made total sense to me and it was maybe the only person that had made a clear decision on their own.

I walked home smiling knowing those simple words made such a powerful impact on me.

I think after being pushed over the edge at work one too many times with being treated unfairly the words I had heard that night had helped give me a clear vision to help me make up my own mind.

It was only then when I walked home from a long day at work that I held my head high and said to myself I was going to London. I had never been so focused on my future, it was the first time I thought about myself for once, what I actually wanted and stop thinking of what other people thought, and best of all, not only did it feel good it felt right.

To this day I still see this friend of mine and although he may not think he's contributed to my career move, he did and with many thanks, I salute him.

The coming weeks brought change, while I was at work my parents were taking time out if their busy schedule to search for a flat for me to rent in London. It was all very exciting but it was equally teeth gritting that I couldn't tell anyone at my current salon what I was planning to do. I also couldn't tell friends just in case it somehow reached the salon.

On the weekends I went down to London on a few occasions to view some flats to see If I liked them but it wasn't all as exciting as I thought it would be.

Any one who has made the jump from their home town to London and rented property will totally understand that when you're almost penniless that there are flats that can, can't and shouldn't ever be lived in. I viewed quiet a few. Some looked nice from the outside but were damp on the inside, some rough some with smashed windows and some that needed a damn good cleaning and I mean gallons of bleach!!!

There were also flats that shouldn't have been

rented out or allowed to be lived in at all, instead they should have been demolished and rebuilt in my opinion.

I kept thinking how on earth some people lived in property like this. It was demoralizing and above all filthy.

I couldn't get my head around the fact that in one house there could be five or move different rooms that were all individually rented out to different people. It felt unsafe and I felt unsure about the whole moving process.

I didn't understand the price of renting, buying or selling, everything was just way out of my league. There's me thinking I was going to move in to a house like my parents had in Derbyshire but how wrong was I?

We eventually came across a flat in a purpose built block, it wasn't actually what I had in mind but to me it felt safe and secure and came at a price that my wage would help in covering the rent although I still had the bills to pay in which my parents helped me out with. Thank-you lovely parents.

It was the first huge step in things to come and it was worth it.

It was Saturday morning and I was at my current salon, I worked all day feeling cagey about all the secrets I had kept away from my so called work mates. I waited until about 5pm and for every body to leave the salon until I handed over my resignation to my manager. Although she was some what surprised I felt that she kind of knew it was going to be happening. She smiled and spoke a few words of courage and friendliness something I hadn't had from any other of the salon staff since I had started my work experience, and with that I made my way through the corridor down the stairs and out of the door taking about ten seconds to glance at myself through the mirror on the wall I had cleaned so many times before. I was on my way home.

Unlike when I was in the London salon there was no need to have that one last tour around the salon nor hang on to the banister on the way out, the last glance in that mirror was enough for me to tell myself I was making the right decision. All the memories were something I didn't really want to keep stored in my mind, I felt I had learned as much as I could in this salon and it was now I had to move on, leave the past behind and start learning real, hardcore hairdressing.

I remember hanging my clothes up on new hangers in my newly rented flat. It was small and basic but it was warm, dry and secure with a kitchen, bathroom, bedroom and a small living room. My parents helped to buy me kitchen utensils a television and the usual home accessories along with what seemed to be a year's supply of tinned food, until I soon found out it wouldn't last long with my appetite.

I started work in the London salon at the beginning of a new month. It was all new to me but I loved it. Different people, new and exiting clients and five star training what more could I ask for? Even the staff liked me. Everyone just seemed to work together and get on.

News travelled fast back in Derbyshire and the local papers where interested in my move to London. It was very strange at first why anyone wanted to know about my decision in career moves but it wasn't everyday a young lad did this kind of thing, landing a potentially successful job in London of all places.

The papers were good to me encouraging and helping me to gain my confidence while being in London without my parents, I was becoming more and more independent and before long I was made head junior to my celebrity stylist boss. Again this was something the papers took interest in and I was asked to continue providing interesting and advisable articles on hairdressing for the next five years, this led also to encouraging other school leavers who wanted to succeed in the hairdressing profession.

I think my mum and dad got a little hassle however it was good, positive hassle after all. People on a daily basis would stop them in the street and ask them if it was their son who kept appearing in the papers and congratulating them as if they too were proud of me even though they hadn't even met me before, but I was so grateful that people were taking an interest after all the shit I had put up with in the early stages of hairdressing, I kept on thinking that surely I did deserved a little something good in return and at last it had come.

I went to work every day setting up equipment and making sure everything was up to standard for my stylist and his clients. These clients were paying around four hundred pound a haircut so I knew it was important to make everything as pristine as possible. Scissors were cleaned and oiled, brushes washed and dried and everything in order to perfection.

Electrical products where lined up in size order along with luxury styling products displaying them whilst reflecting in front of the mirror. I was working alongside my mentor and was being trained one to one every day in the salon. I felt the luckiest boy on earth.

From the day I had watched another junior setting up the equipment it was now my turn to impress my mentor and I was going to try much harder than I had ever tried before.

I was so enthusiastic I used to watch every move the boss used to make, in my eyes I was studying the best hairdresser in London and even the UK.

I knew the more I watched the more I learnt and the more I learnt the better I became.

I started to sequence every move he made so much so I could visualize the technique over and over in my head knowing what his next move would be and what section he was going to take next.

I trained in the evenings learning not only the art of hairdressing but the way to visualize shape and style. I was learning the master's knowledge.

It became a kind of obsession with noting down in my mind his every move and his every angle, I knew I had become fascinated with his way of working and I was soon characterizing his movements not only in his work but also at home.

I started to recognize his dress sense his stance his routines and his general well being and aura.

It was at this point that many people were telling me I had become his prodigy and the more I heard it being said the more I obsessed on studying his ways and means of hairdressing.

We worked closely day to day and we got to know the ins and outs of each other as they say, however there was something else that I had also found out, something that I knew was true but because I idolized this guy so much I tried so hard to push it to the back of my memory. I didn't want to believe but I really knew it was true, as I saw things a boy my age should never have seen.

On many occasions as much as we got on I was also in the firing line if things didn't go his way or to plan.

He often flew in to rages, rages that were so upsetting for me to be involved in that on many occasions I would often just find myself taking the blame for things that weren't actually my fault just to get through the issue. When I say the word rage I'm talking eyes of anger and red chest and neck being able to see the anger rising up his face. It may sound harsh but that is the only way to explain it.

Not many people saw these disruptions they

were mainly outside of work, in the car on the way home or at home itself.

I didn't quite understand these temper tantrums as one minute we could be at his home having dinner having a laugh and the next he would go in to one. How could someone be so polite one minute and then so evil and nasty the next? At one point after learning everything from him I felt I knew nothing. He became someone who could make you feel a million dollars one minute or worthless the next. I didn't understand and it didn't make sense.

The thing was, everyone was so interested in me working with this hairdresser genius that I found it hard to say anything bad about him as deep down inside I totally understood his theory and philosophy on hair, I felt that I would not only let myself down but also so many other people if I spoke the truth.

One day we had a photo shoot at the salon, the camera crew had turned up as had the models for the day and also the makeup artist and wardrobe, the only thing missing was the boss.

I was asked several times if I knew where he was by the crew but I hadn't seen him all morning. Time was moving on and yet the boss had still not turned up for the shoot.

We waited and waited but to no avail of his appearance. It was then I was told by the salon manager to go to his house to get him.

I arrived at the house a short taxi journey away from the salon where I was met by another driver explaining that he had been waiting to pick the boss up three hours ago but he found him not to be in.

I knocked on the door and then rang the bell but there was no response. I tried looking through the letter box however it just seemed to be an empty shell of a house.

It dawned on me to grasp the door handle and turn it not thinking about breaking and entering but the door did move and open so I cautiously entered being extremely quiet for some reason.

I checked the downstairs rooms. When I entered the first room I was completely shocked, it was full of cd's and dvd's all over the floor and what looked like paper work all over the place. It didn't even look like the same house. I walked in to the kitchen to a mess of spilt wine and food, rubbish piled up in corner after corner overflowing bins and the smell of stale alcohol. I couldn't believe my eyes.

On the side was white powder as if like baking flour or talcum powder, it was everywhere, yet some had been left on cookery books or on the worktops in a long line fashion.

Things started to sink in, I had heard from so many of the staff at the salon about the problems the boss was facing, the problems that were destroying him and now I had come face to face with the reality of seeing it for myself with my own eyes. I was heartbroken to think that all I had heard and all the rumors where actually a reality.

The truth had hit me hard, I stood in the kitchen with no thought of anything just a distant glare at the white lines counting each of them as I scanned the room, it was then that I heard footsteps coming down the stairs, it was the boss. I greeted him and soon turned on my work mode explaining about the shoot and that he was extremely late, I watched him as he struggled turning his t-shirt inside out for no apparent reason, in fact he didn't even know his head from his arse if I'm to be honest. He struggled concentrating on what I was saying and couldn't focus his eyes on me at all, I knew myself he didn't actually know where he was or what the hell he was doing, all he said was for me to go back to the salon and he would meet me there. I did what he said as his behavior was slowly becoming more and more uncontrollable, I jumped in the cab and made my way back to the salon.

In the cab I couldn't stop myself from thinking about what I had seen, I was so upset inside but more than anything I was hurt. To see and know my mentor in that kind of state was utterly shocking.

When I was working alongside him it felt good and it felt right but there was one thing I just couldn't become, one thing I didn't want to learn and one thing I never wanted to follow and that was to become an addict.

I sat in the cab racking my brain over what I was going to tell the manager and the crew, trying to find a way which I thought would be right but I changed my story so many times I even baffled myself with what I wanted to say, I also didn't want to loose my job so I took the chance of keeping stum and saying that he would meet back at the salon very soon.

That day he never did turn up for the photo shoot. Disappointment all round, I felt stupid. I felt angry and worst of all I felt humiliated.

I know it sounds sad or self absorbed or almost stalker like but I really wanted this opportunity, I changed my presence to which I was back home and with working with a wealthy clientele I learnt to grow up much more quickly and take responsibilities and situations in my stride. I was looked upon with great respect and people praised my every move, the best thing was there was never any jealousy it was all done with good intentions.

I loved my job and I loved the position I was in however whenever I was alone which was normally once I got home to my rented flat after work, I often had a little cry to myself thinking about what I had seen that day in the bosses house, it bothered me knowing I had changed so much to be like my mentor and he had let me down. This also led on to thinking about being here on my own and having no mum or dad with me by my side. I had some lonely times in London but I always kept those times to myself. It was breaking my heart being away from home yet I knew I was doing much more and much better here in London than I ever would have if I was back home.

I've now learnt to be independent for myself and I still think about my family every day. Not one day goes by when I don't.

Many people say that London can be a very lonely place at times and I can assure you I have had my fair share of feeling alone. I have been lucky enough to have met so many people throughout my life that maybe to this day still have no idea how much they have kept me feeling up beat about myself when I have been feeling at my lowest.

The two guys dressed in green suits outside the members club opposite Berkley Square, staff from the Mayfair hotels that I am so lucky to be friends of (you know who you all are) the security guard I very often walked past on the way to work standing outside one of the Embassy's overlooking Grosvenor Square and the friends I've made in the wine bar on Mount Street, you have all made a huge impact on me in some shape or form without your knowing. I strongly appreciate you all.

I don't want to sober on about emotional stuff but I'll put it in my acknowledgements so make sure you read it!!!

I was twenty one when I sat in my bosses car on the way back from a long day in the studio having a very normal chat about work in the salon, when he asked me how I thought I was getting on in my training? I thought at the time it was a very odd question to ask me as it was him who was training me in the first place and if any one should know it should have been him, but as he asked me and therefore I told him how I felt. I felt I was ready to qualify as a stylist but hey, I may have been a little bias.

All I really wanted to ask was about that

disturbing day I witnessed but I kept my mouth closed and just answered the question.

We arrived back at the salon and dropped off the equipment. We walked upstairs to the first floor and he went in to the toilet, it was then he called me to the bathroom. He asked me if I had been happy with my work as I stood in the door frame of the toilet, an odd place to have this conversation. He continued to ask if I had all my own equipment.

He was vague in his questions and didn't really seem to be that concerned however he was becoming increasingly more agitated trying to find something that seemed to be lost in his jacket pocket.

Shortly within time after finding the small square piece of paper he was so desperately looking for he said "congratulations, you start work on Monday morning as a stylist".

I was so amazed, this guy I so admired had told me I was ready and believe me I was ready, roll on Monday morning. I walked away happy at what he had said to me however equally in dismay as I knew he was going to be doing something that I knew wasn't right either, as these pieces of small white folded up pieces of paper were the disgusting evidence of the killer habit which I had seen so many times before, but hey, I heard what I had needed to and wanted to hear.

Within time I worked my self up the ladder becoming a stylist, from junior stylist to designer stylist onwards and upwards. I felt I had achieved what I had set out for.

I was a busy stylist once I had built up my clientele and when my boss was away on holiday or out of the salon his clients started to come and see me, it had become like a new venture, a new way of wiping the slate clean, I was privileged to be working here but this time as a qualified stylist.

Many days I was recommended clients not only from the receptionists but from the man himself.

I learnt to be able to draw my hairstyles before I had even cut the hair just like he did, it wasn't just about holding a pair of scissors but the whole package of service, being able to consult clients in a much more professional manner meant the service became more personal and bespoke for everyone.

We went from photo shoots and TV appearances to magazine articles all in one day. The diary was fully booked and I met and worked with celebrities, TV personalities, royalty, footballers and pop singers on a regular basis. It was fab. The only thing was, my boss had a strange habit of wondering off from time to time often to the toilet. Strange as it was it wasn't long until it clicked that his habit was becoming more clear to me but it was something that I couldn't get my head around as his actions made him become more and more obvious about the whole thing.

From the day I was sitting on the receptions sofa sweating nervously I was now working as a qualified stylist all my dreams had come true. I recommended and sold products, provided consultations and introduced colour to my clientele, I was doing what every good stylist was doing at the salon, I felt that I had made it in the hairdressing world only to be slightly disappointed that my boss didn't seem to share the same enthusiasm, he was so up and down he didn't seem to really care yet I thought he would have been proud of me as he trained me and successfully invented a new prodigy of himself.

The days flew by although they were extremely long hours.

I found myself most evenings in the salon alone as I was ever increasing my new clientele.

I kept pushing and pushing to be the best, overtaking stylists that had been at the salon for years on their price brackets.

The boss and I still worked alongside each other everyday. Although he never patted me on the back or asked me how I was getting on I was still very proud to be working there.

He always recommended his clients to me and also when ever he was on holiday the clients were often booked over to myself.

I remember being booked a client, a gent that was smartly dressed and well spoken and before we began to talk about his hair he told me a story.

He attended an event which my boss had also attended and whilst there he payed a visit to the bathroom. Whilst standing doing his business my boss also visited the bathroom and took his stance next to this client.

The client turned and looked at my boss and

instantly recognized him, as strange as it may seem he discussed with my boss that his hair cut was done with myself at his salon. My boss seemed pretty impressed and after hearing this story I felt for once that my boss did actually realize the work I was putting in especially with such a good repour from a client, even if it was in unusual circumstances.

After around 10 years at the salon cracks in the boss started to slowly appear. The tantrums and trauma's became to worsen and this was only the start.

The little things that I had seen before about the bosses' actions other people were also noticing. It was only then I could see the dangers of what was becoming of the main man himself and the start of the down turn of the success he once had.

On many occasions clients would book appointments with him around 11am yet to find that they would be kept waiting as he was either running late or hadn't even left the house. This normally meant that he hadn't woke up. The most common excuse was the stuck in traffic gag. Some clients would wait two or maybe three hours to then be told by an extremely embarrassed and apologetic receptionist that they would have to reschedule their appointment as a matter of urgency had come up and the boss wouldn't be in to cut their hair. But we knew there wasn't any urgency, for all we knew he may not have even arrived home from the night before. Whatever the reasons we kept it quiet as it was the most subtle way to let the clients down. However, there was never a right way.

It soon became natural for this to be a regular routine of events.

It also started to affect the staff and other salon clients.

They always say that responsibility and punctuality starts from the top so it was no surprise when other stylist started to take less pride in their work and arrive late too.

Once this takes place it seemed to also rub off on to the younger assistants, they too were taking the whole lead by example to a whole new level.

Seeing him like this was devastating for me let alone everyone else. He became more and more vacant from the salon and his staff. Although I spoke to him he often seemed away from the conversation sometimes making you feel like he wasn't even listening to what you had to say.

His eyes were often glazed and his style started to become unkempt.

I had never seen him like this before. It was scary. He was scary.

When he was in the salon his demands became more inappropriate, his rages more often which led to anyone crossing him would put themselves in the line of being fired or a very organized constructive dismissal. Staff started to keep themselves away from him to save their own job security.

Talk in the salon was becoming negative and the stylists started to lose their moral and interest not only in the salon but also their in their own work. After all if you have no one to look up to then what's the point? You can't blame the stylists for how they were acting either as their boss was the culprit within the beginning of the down fall of the salon.

The running of the salon also became increasingly worse. He would often over ride decisions and not listen to others that were trying to help. This not only created a bad vibe but staff also started falling out with each other and the last thing you want to do is upset a bunch of egotistic hairdressers wielding scissors and hairdryers.

Rumor, speculation, truth or untrue remarks, word began to circulate around the salon and soon it had become known to other salons in the area that the boss had a personal addiction.

For all those years we had all known of the problems although it was now out in the open. You know things are bad when clients even tell you that they had read things in newspapers about his out of hand, known reputation.

It hurt like hell, my heart had given up and I had also lost respect.

I think in life you can try and try and try to help someone, but when somebody doesn't help themselves then you will always be fighting a losing battle.

It was a very sad time for me. Not only was I working with a hairdressing great he had let me down with his behavior and personal issues and everybody knew. I felt embarrassed.

To walk in the restroom of the salon to face a white powdery surface, a mixture of powder and crumbling crumbs of the highly addictive substance made me sick, I could only think that if I was walking in on this so many times how many clients where doing the same?

Although he occasionally came in to work to do clients he often spent more time in the toilets in between clients which made him run behind on appointments. This upset clients with waiting and also not getting the haircuts they expected. More and more complaints came in and less and less staff wanted to deal with angry clients on a day to day basis.

I too was trying desperately to keep my clients happy with all the issues arising in the background.

They asked me questions about recent tabloid issues in which I had given up lying to protect him and could only tell the truth, and then the day came that made me clear my mind of all negatives and put me back on track. Thank god it was said to me as this was the day that changed my life!!!!!!

A client came in to see me. I had my consultation, washed her hair and sat down to start cutting when she told me that this would be her last time that she would be visiting the salon.

It was devastating to hear however as you'd expect with instinct I asked why. The answer and the exact wording was " I am not going to keep putting money through his till and lining his pockets to keep feeding his habit"!!!

She had been coming to the salon for over 10 years and explained she had seen lots of changes. In all those years the boss had never once said hello to her although he had walked past her almost every time she had been to the salon.

I could sympathize with her but hang on, although I was agreeing with her I was also losing a client.

Many clients had said the same to me in a round about way however it was me who was being stung for it.

I understood their theory but it was affecting me also, they were my livelihood, I cared about my clients, my clients were like my best friends.

I waited for days to try and catch the boss in what I thought would be one of his better, good mood days so I could approach him to discuss the delicate issues that was affecting the salon, sadly however it turned out to be the wrong day!!!!!!One word.................. RAGE!!!!!!!!!!!

The language was appalling, I was in shock when he told me that if I thought I could run a salon better than him then I should go ahead and open a salon myself. He continued, he was the godfather of hairdressing and that he is the best hairdresser of all time, he told people what to do and know one tells him what to do. I felt sick, I was trying to help, I just thought he needed to know, I wasn't an addict, I wasn't the one on drugs,,,,,,,,,,,,I WAS BETTER THAN HIM!

Days went by thinking about what my client had said and more and more complaints came in to the salon regarding the service, expense and cleanliness. I didn't want to be part of this mess, all I wanted to do was to provide the best service I could possibly give. I think I was thinking on behalf of the majority of the staff too.

I stood watching from a corner of the salon as mistakes where being made and the salon moral was defiantly deflating.

Clients, stylists and juniors looked unhappy, the atmosphere was distant and the overall efficiency of the salon was lacking. This wasn't the salon I worked in as a seventeen year old. Back then it was electric, now depressing.

I had now taken it upon myself to start making decisions to try and help put him back on the right path in the hairdressing industry regardless to the foul mouthed argument he threw at me.

As time went by I started making notes and decisions about the salon and once I'd done my homework I made the vital call to the salon owner.

The salon owner was not the boss, it was the bosses ex partner, although they always publicized the fact they work together in business it was more a media stunt to save explanation and embarrassment however away from the media they hated and despised each other often competing against each other spoiling there children to pick up the favorite or who's the best parent badge?

Although she so called 'ran' the salon the partner was far more interested purely in the money side of things, an obsession she couldn't hide or keep to herself, it was more like the old saying, give her enough rope and eventually,,,,, the rest you can decide what happens.

I was soon sat around the partners house with

my dad drinking tea served by one of her many house keepers. It was all a little too pretentious to be honest but hey, she seemed a lonely women who didn't seem to have many true friends so I m guessing the house keepers helped to keep her company day to day. Me and my dad would have been happy discussing this in a local pub. My dads often said that most business has been done in pubs over a few beers. I believe him.

We discussed the problems with the salon as I sat there opening up about what I thought were the solutions.

We talked endlessly about what should be done and also if I could invest in the salon to help move the brand onwards and upwards and to help get my boss the help that he really needed.

She nervously told us both that she was always known for being the successful business women out of herself and the boss, and made it clear that she liked to use the story of herself running the salon empire and the boss just doing the hair bit but if it wasn't for her it wouldn't be a success. But she was soon to contradict herself by saying that they used a lot of these storylines to help headline the media and their success was down to little more that luck, suing people and a stock room full of bullshit which really did make more sense.

After much discussion the three of us came up with a mutual decision that it would be a great idea to get on board, so another meeting with her accountant was penciled in the book for the following week before she fashionably squeezed in a celebrity name to name drop she had to go and see after we had left. She was a woman who never really lived in the real world and always made you feel that she was more superior than yourself, but when I've had the time to look back at the situation I think it was more a case that she should have been extremely honored and lucky that I had ever introduced her to my dad in the first place.

We walked into the boardroom to meet their accountants. There was a large, long, old wooden table which around sat about eight chairs, the uncomfortable chairs you usually find in any boardroom. Every one of importance came busily into the room and took their seats ready to discuss the investment process further. We looked through spreadsheets and accounts for the previous years, to be honest, I didn't really know myself what all the figures meant I was just pleased that my father was sat beside me. However it wasn't long before we had started talking about sharing views delving deeper and deeper into endless numbers, lines, charts and graphs.

My father has always been very knowledgeable in this kind of field after running his own business for many years, listening to my dad kept me at ease as I noticed the accountants sitting opposite nervously, constantly moving, gradually becoming more agitated as my father fired question after question across the table.

There were two accountants opposite myself and my dad, I can always remember seeing them constantly looking at one another as if to look for a response, answer or suggestion from each other when answering questions from our side. And then, the most vital piece of information made the pieces of the jigsaw fall into place. The words "don't invest" were spoken.

"Don't invest in this business as the books are not true to their figures". We both sat in a mixture of amazement and shock as they went on. They reeled off all the reasons as to why we should not invest in the company, I couldn't believe I had been working for almost fourteen years alongside one of London's so called greatest hairdressers, after all the media coverage he had built up and the time he had owned his salon, he was in such financial danger.

The constant words of his empire and achievements along with the amount of times he used to tell me how much he was worth only to find out he hadn't always told me the truth. My mind was rolling over and over about all the things that he used to say to me and it was only now I was wondering how much he had told me could have been all a fabrication of lies.

I couldn't keep up with the conversation in the room it was all too much for me to hear all the problems they were having with the salon due to the boss. Secretly I was holding back my disappointment and feeling very emotional, I felt as though I had been led on for the last fourteen years, following a fake. For the very first time it made sense to me that the run of success this man had achieved was merely based on past glorified opportunities. The fast car, house and boastful performances around women were all bullshit and most worrying of all, everything was on credit.

The meeting was drawn to a swift yet embarrassing end, not only for myself but also for the nervous accountants, I think they knew all along the seriousness of the investment and although they were working for the salon even they couldn't bring themselves to see this investment go through to help the ever worryingly sinking ship. I must thank them for their honesty, however I felt more sorry for them having lived a lie for so many years and working on behalf of such selfish, ignorant and greedy individuals.

It was then I realized I had to move on away from the salon and the thought of going it alone became more and more appealing to me, but how? How on earth could I afford to do this? Not only that but I had never even though of leaving where I was, after all, I had always thought I was generally happy working for the mentor that had seriously let me down.

Weeks went by trying to find the right day to catch my boss in a good enough mood to talk about the meeting I had with his accountants in the most sensitive way possible, as I knew he was prone to outrageous primadonna rages. And in time I found the day to pick my moment.

We were soon sat talking over margarita cocktails in his lounge one evening. We spoke about the salon and the staff and also about his personal life which I had not expected to be brought up in conversation, yet every time we reached the subject of the meeting he seemed to scarper away out of the room not really saying where he was going yet re-appearing a little worse for wear on his arrival back to the sofa. The conversation started to become personal but not between the both of us but about his staff, people he didn't want working there and how he was going to find a way of letting them go without having to fire them, but all I was here for was to discuss my meeting with his people.

I listened patiently trying to edge in on what I was here for but unfortunately to no avail, the more cocktails we drank the later it became and the more frequent he was leaving the room ten minutes at a time, each time seemingly to worsen his speech his focus all around the room sniffing profusely.

As it was getting late I thought it was time to make my move and tell him my thoughts about my future, as you can imagine it wasn't successful and I had to listen to an aggressive, tanked up guy for yet another couple of hours when all I wanted to do at this point was go home.

It was around 1am when I decided I had to do or say something so I could leave the house and head home. The atmosphere had fallen and an evil surrounding had set in, although yet again he was out the room and upstairs doing his thing however when he entered the lounge this time not only was he all over the place he came in to the room as if nothing had happened, no fall out no rage and no hard feelings only one other thing that I couldn't believe I was seeing. I wasn't going to write this in the book although after serious thought I took it upon myself to always keep this book real and tell it how it is, after all the things I have gone through and all the things I put up with that I never deserved I think its only fair, so here goes…….

He sat on the sofa crossed legged still slurping the margarita whilst sniffing away. He was wearing a white untucked shirt with white linen trousers, but not for long.

I always knew he had a problem but to actually see his white linens from waist to knee suddenly turn to a nasty wet orange colour I was horrified and embarrassed for him.

It was a sad sight to see yet he sat there as if nothing had happened as he carried on talking shit.

I sat for a minute stunned, he looked lonely, disheveled, tired and old and there was nothing I could do but say goodbye and close the door behind me. I stood outside the house and called a cab wishing that this night had not even taken place.

I know it may sound selfish but I too had given up on him and now I totally understood why other people said the things they did about him. He didn't care about anyone, all he did care about was when he was taking his next fix. People like this really do need help but unfortunately I'm not one of these people who can help with these matters.

After witnessing a bizarre evening, once I was on my way home in the cab all I could think about was whether or not he was still alive as I had left him in a state irresponsibly.

Over the next few weeks I started wandering the

streets of Mayfair searching for anywhere that displayed a 'To let' sign outside. Each day after work I would walk the streets an extra couple of hours seeing what property there was in the area, but every evening was more disappointing as everything for rent was either a first floor office or basement, it was so frustrating as I was looking for a ground floor shop with a shop front.

I viewed everything I could and after endless searching I soon found that many of the estate agents didn't take me serious or didn't have time for me, I had the impression that they were use to working with the big Mayfair boys not a young guy like myself who was a hairdresser, but I was focused enough to be stubborn and stand my ground and within the following few months I had found a property to put down a secured deposit to start the beginning of my hairdressing career.

Christmas was ever nearing and a cold empty shop in Mayfair was beginning to take shape.

I worked in the salon telling know one of the eruption that was between the boss and myself.

I kept silent.

Christmas in the salon was quiet, it wasn't the same as most years as the salon had lost many clients due to bad management, high turnover of staff and overall lack of customer care.

I tried not to let it bother me too much as I was quietly perusing my own dreams.

I started back to work after Christmas my notice in my pocket ready to hand in to the manager.

I wasn't nervous as I'd had a long time to think over my decisions and I knew I was making the right one.

After talking to one or two stylist friends of mine word was soon creating a lively environment and so sooner than later I handed in my notice and left the salon.

Whilst walking out the salon doors at 5.30pm I knew immediately I had made the right decision, I took one last grip of the salons wearing door knob and opened it slowly. I turned to face the salon this one last time as a few memories flashed back over the last few years, I let the door slowly close behind me and never looked back. I walked up to the new salon being carful to make sure know one was following me and got myself changed in to some old clothes to help my dad with the refit of the salon as we hadn't much time, we was opening the following Tuesday

In the next week we had kitted the salon out and turned a run down ground floor and basement in to a luxury, boutique five star hair salon. With a little help from some friends in Derbyshire I must say we had done a great job. You really do find out who your friends are when you really need them. I had heard nothing from the ex boss so I seemed to think he actually didn't care about the loss of one of his positive high earning stylists.

What came next was totally unplanned and overwhelming, within days of leaving over four hundred clients had called up the previous salon to book appointments with me only to be told I was no longer working there. Not only had the reception team told the clients where I was but many of my ex colleagues had told them of my where abouts too. Clients also searched the internet to find me as they wanted to be booked in for their hair to be styled by myself and my team at my new salon and just to add to further the excitement, other stylists had also left on hearing my departure and had asked to work with me. Of Course this was a great pleasure in the greatest respect that they had in wanting to come with me, the belief in me and the trust in me. Thanks guys.

We opened our doors on January 11th as I remember the day was 11/01/11, all the one's and within the first week the phones became jammed with the amount of calls being taken for bookings. It was great to see clients walking through our very own salon doors and the running of the salon was perfect.

We served every client with complimentary refreshments and head massages, everyone was on a high from the excitement and I was thrilled to say the least. My mobile would constantly vibrate with messages from friends and family congratulating myself and the staff on our successful opening until I answered my mobile phone to a well known number I was unfortunate to forget about, it was the ex boss.

I knew a conversation was going to be on the cards but I had no idea what was coming my way.

I can assure you it wasn't a friendly conversation neither a chat about success but more about a screaming and shouting match mainly from his mouth. The language was yet again appallingly disgusting, threatening behavior, in a way it was a form of bullying or harassment somewhat controlling however I'm not sure that when someone says that they will close your newly opened business down or break your wrists to stop you from being able to work is actually illegal, but it certainly was a major scare tactic and I'm not to big or proud to say that I was at that moment concerned for my wellbeing.

He also brought up that he wanted me to pay a hefty sum of money to him as compensation for what income I would have made for him if I'd had stayed working for him that year. None of this made sense to me, I remembered the day he said to me that if I thought it was easy opening a salon then go ahead and do it, and that's exactly what I did and now he was giving me verbal abuse for doing so. It was his idea in the first place!!!

My parents were also mentioned in the conversation, however, I have been brought up to have manners and to be better to take higher ground as not to talk about them as he did. I would never stray so low to do that to anyone, neither would I talk so disrespectful of his parents, nor do I want to harm anyone's family.

My ex bosses threatening behavior raised my awareness as to how he had gained such a ghastly vendetta against me. It wasn't about the salon or the staff that followed me, it was about me and only me, more about proving a point as I had heard over the phone how he always won court cases as he was the hairdressing genius and know one will ever be as good as he in the industry.

He also described how he would help me lose my house and salon and that he would in time stop me from doing hairdressing ever again, it was one of the worst moments in my life.

The call was left with a threatening message to take me to court and the phone line cut off.

Days later I was summoned a letter to attend court.

I was ordered a court summons and was soon being sued by the ex boss.

I always knew it was going to be more of a vendetta towards me than anything else however we went to court to face the music.

I was annoyed at the fact that this had happened and that he had wanted to take things this far. None of this made sense. It was just as if he wanted me to open my own salon so he could sue me all along, as if planned. All I could think about was the drugs he was taking and maybe it was partly the cause to help him make money and help him out on the salon debt and problems.

I sat in the concrete corridor inside the court feeling not just cold and empty but angry as I could see the opposition at the other end of the long stone hall, all I wanted to do was go to work yet they were trying all they could to close me down and stop me.

The day was long and frustrating back and forth with negotiations from each side but everything that they wanted I disagreed on, whether it was about money or trading I was not going to be put in a situation where I felt I was being either bullied in to or not making an agreement on my terms. I could see that the more I declined or disagreed the more agitated the other side seemed to react and because the boss never attended court, each time I sent over my solicitor they had to make a phone call to the boss to ask him what he wanted to do next. It eventually came to a point where I didn't think that even he actually knew what he was doing.

I stared up towards the clock, it was around 2pm and we were still no where near in making a decision to negotiate, myself and the team sitting quietly around the table. The time had come and the judge was ready for us to sit in the court room to fight this mess out once and for all. I was ready to stand my corner no matter what, I wanted to work I was proud to work and know one was going to stop me.

The boss never turned up for court which I cant really sit here and say made it easier as I'd like to of done this face to face as I worked everyday looking at my clients through a mirror and I was use to talking to people directly, but everyday he never made an appearance and to be honest I wished I wasn't sat here in the first place. I can sometime understand why there are people in the world not wanting to work as there always seems to be someone out there trying to constantly bring you down.

We all took our places in the court room and I was sitting directly behind the representatives the ex boss had fronted for bringing me down. Thinking about it, if I could give any advice for their side I think I would have found a rep that at least looked as though they wanted to be there but they couldn't have looked further from their comfort zone and so far away from knowing what they were saying. In fact, they had no idea.

It seemed as if everything they said the judge had lots of reasons to question them, many of those questions being about why they wanted to stop me from trading and what was to gain if they achieved the result they desperately wanted. It merely felt as if there really wasn't a case at all, however they continued to push their case while I sat quietly listening to all the false sentences they were saying about me.

Let me take this time to tell you that before you go in to court you say and sign a kind of clause to say that you speak the truth the whole truth and nothing but the truth, only I was telling the truth, I didn't have a story to tell or to lie about I was here just to give my side of events, not to 'out-do' or get one over on anyone but I couldn't believe what I was hearing. The only thing I was thinking was how on earth were 'they' allowed to lie? Lies, lies, lies.

It crossed my mind several times as to why it had even made it this far, I couldn't believe after fifteen years of going to work everyday and not being late once, staying behind after hours and always going the extra mile why he was doing this to me?

In time it was my solicitor's opportunity to

stand and speak my ground.

To cut a long story short we had nothing to lie about and they told it how it was.

We were told to rise and the judge disappeared through a door nearby. We sat in silence.

About fifteen minutes later we rose again and the judge took her place in the center of the room, we all took our seats and she began explaining what was going to happen next.

I wasn't sure what I was expecting but at least an answer would have been nice, however the case was adjourned until a further week so the judge could read through the case and make a decision before we went to trial. We left the court room and discussed further processes with my solicitor before walking out on to the busy street and back in to the world of normality. I wasn't happy neither sad, it was a long day of talks but I felt like I had achieved nothing.

The opposition stood confused at the outcome, although they appeared to not want to be there, they also were the puppets for the day.

A week later I had received a letter to say that the court date was set and the case was heading for trial.

It was a shame, but there was nothing I could do but get myself ready, focused and my mind straight.

All the pressure of getting a salon together in time for opening and now a high court trial over a hairdressing salon, it had almost become a handbags drawn scenario.

Without going in to too much and also the fact of legal reasons I can tell you that after waiting a week for the trial that was to cause an awful lot of unnecessary worrying and stress, he had called my solicitors to say he wanted to pull out and WE WON THE CASE, nothing to do with the in-between phone call to me with yet another threatening message. I think that was the call that made him realize he had made a huge mistake once the phone line went down. I think he realized I was standing my ground through thick and thin and I was happy for it to be settled in court. He on the other hand wasn't.

I didn't have time to be joyful even though we won the case.

In situations like these it comes to affect not only myself and the team but also your family and friends. Sometimes people can become down seeing others not acting their usual selves and the same had happened to us and the people around us. It wasn't something I was excited about, it wasn't about being the winner it was about getting on with the salon and being there for my staff and for my clients.

It was pathetic after all, and although I may seem a little bias but when over a hundred people are telling you the same you do start to think that maybe it wasn't me but it was him that was bitter about the whole thing. It seemed we had walked out of court and carried on working, what a load of stress for nothing, only it didn't end there.

Not only had he pulled out and lost the case his

anger and bitterness would get the better of him. He wasn't happy at the fact that for maybe the very first time in his career he couldn't be given what he asked for. He was use to shouting orders and making demands, he was use to getting what he wanted but this time he had failed so he asked the courts for an injunction to be put on myself and the staff instead of closing me down.

It was something that was so very petty to go through with such an extreme procedure that even words fail me to this day.

No-one in the right mind would ever steep so low, however, I guess he was rarely in the right mind.

An injunction to not deal with any of our previous clients for a period of time and also not to employ any ex staff I had previously worked with for six months to give him the chance to try to maintain the four hundred clients that had already left his salon to start a fresh in ours.

People wanted change, people wanted a different environment where customer care and loyalty played a huge part.

I very often look back and think that these injunctions especially for hairdressers and for people in these circumstances should never be allowed.

Not only do you take the jump in to opening your own business but when you do you can't do your clients. Which in theory limits your trade, and when you have rents, rates, wages and bills to pay this is a heavy restriction to accept.

I have totally lost all interest and respect of my

ex boss, I didn't care about the personal problems he had or either the problems he was having with his salon, it was clear to me that his ex partner was only in the business for one thing and he needed to keep up with his ongoing habit.

To have to tell your clients that you can't do their hair seems so wrong, a little embarrassing even, but when you have friends and clients that understand, believe in you, wait and be patient with you, above all they will become loyal to you too.

We operated our salon only taking on brand new clients for the first half of the year. I was a little worried the fact that having over four hundred phone calls within the first week or so I now couldn't continue to do their hair for the next six months. I was devastated. We were lucky we were in a busy area of Mayfair and thankfully we were doing well with passing trade and creating business with other local businesses.

In the hairdressing business nothing can be kept quiet. Hairdressers chat world wide with other stylist and salons and word can get round in no time at all. It's kind of like a hairdressing network, a face book of hairdressers connecting and sharing ideas and gossip.

The injunction soon became general knowledge within the hairdressing community spreading not only from salon to salon but from shops to banks to offices and cafes within the area. The clients that we were turning away from the salon were talking of the disgust that someone could have stooped so low to do this to myself and my team. I thought at first it was going to be myself that would get the back lash of unhappy clients telling me they were massively pissed off but it seemed apparent that it wasn't myself but my ex employer that was receiving the back lash as clients where entering his salon and complaining.

Cabbies were also talking about us to their customers as they were going about their day to day business. The word was out and the word was on the streets, up in the buildings above and below let alone across the internet.

It also helped as we were still friends with many hairdressers from the previous salon.

Many of these stylists would openly tell their clients where we had opened and also passed our details on to them. Without us having to do any PR at all it seemed as if they were doing our entire PR for us recommending their own clients to our salon. I knew it didn't make sense but I wasn't going to stop the majority of their staff from doing me free advertisement.

I was even told by clients that they had called to make an appointment with me at the previous salon to be told that I was no longer there however the receptionists would also tell of our where a-bouts.

I was being advertised everyday by their salon that had originally put the injunction on me in the first place. I was being groomed to perfection without breaking any of the injunctions myself and it felt great!

Clients would come in to our shop understanding the injunction but would pop in anyway to let us know they would be back to see us in six months time. This was a great feeling knowing that these people were not just clients but friends. Real friends.

Ex staff also came in to the salon on a day to day basis telling us about how the atmosphere in their salon had worsened and how appalled they were at what their boss had done to us.

I couldn't believe the comments they were saying however they kept working there for him. I have soon learnt that some people have an awful lot of big talk, but unfortunately no balls to go ahead with the ideas that come from their mouth. I strongly recommend not saying anything if you're not going to follow things through, it's a very strong comment to make but always think before you speak otherwise you could one day make a comment that some day you may regret.

It also became noticeable that the majority of the staff at the previous salon were extremely unhappy in their work place, however, I must say how hard it is to explain that its not until you leave you realize the opportunities that are out there and that you don't need to put up with the nonsense that you have put up with for such a long time if you don't need to. Life's short.

On July 11th our injunction ended and we were free to open our salon doors to our regular clients.

For anyone thinking of opening their own salon let me tell you now so you know not to feel let down that not all of your regular clients will follow you. Unfortunately I found that the clients throughout your career that always say they will follow you know matter where you go don't always stand up to their word. Although at first it was disheartening I have learnt to accept that you can't please everyone but after long thought I know for sure that the service we provide in our salon is excellent at an affordable tariff, so if some people feel happier paying much more money for less service and talent then it's all good by me. We welcome the fact that there are so many salons around and more and more people are finding more confidence walking in to hair salons which I think is great. We hope even more people come and visit us as you are not forgotten about, we hope to be your official hair salon some day soon.

Work began building up our clientele and the clients came in thick and fast, it was an exciting time for all the team and a chance to provide our clients with the best possible service they have ever received.

We didn't dwell on the past talking about the experience we had been through however I promised myself I would write a book to put the record straight in my very own words for all to read.

I hope you enjoy.

Since renting a flat in London and barely being able to afford to pay my rent, I have now learnt the achievement of success.

As for the injunction in my own words, everyone

should have the right to learn, everyone should have the right to educate others, everyone should have the right to become successful and move forward and everyone should have the right to open a new business being able to trade.

Most importantly everyone should be able to follow their dreams.

Whilst writing this book I am still working at our salon in London's Mayfair everyday.

I am now proud to say I am officially a salon owner and I run a busy column of clients on a day to day basis, including involving all my team in photo shoots, session work, catwalk shows and events.

I am heavily involved in the ongoing five star training of our staff and follow the progression of the younger talent of up and coming juniors and junior stylists.

My clients include high profile business men and women, celebrities and royals. It's all part of the job.

Why is it when you work as a hairstylist you never get chance to ever get your own hair cut?

Also, why are your parents always the last to ever get there hair done when they really should come first?

So what makes us different? Well, many companies recommend never mixing business with pleasure and that's where I'm afraid to say I disagree. My clients are not just clients they are friends, and I hope the feeling has become mutual. That's what makes our salon different. We care about the people we deal with, not just over an appointment or when they re-book with us but also when they leave our salon. I like to think we are their personal stylist and whenever they need me or my team we are always there.

Thank you to you all.

And finally, thank you to hairdressing for providing me with the talent and skill I am so thankful to obtain and also to all of the clients who have let me cut their hair over the past years, I really appreciate your kindness and support. I hope to cut many different styles on all of you in the years to come and keep you all up to date in the world of fashion. We are here to attend to all your hair needs and requirements.

I have said so many times to my clients that I have learnt more from the people who have sat in my chair having a hair cut than I have around a board room table, so a huge Thank-you goes out to all that have helped guide me and understand me.

You have all made my dream come true. Thank you.

Acknowledgments

I have made many mistakes in my life and I'm sure many more will follow from which I will learn from using the advice and ideas from the team that have always stood by me.

I've taken criticism, jealousy and bullying on the chin but with time I have learnt to become stronger and to keep trying.

At times when I have felt lonely and alone a phone call which feels a million miles away can regain faith and safety in an incredible millisecond.

If it wasn't for an old manuscript being accidentally read by a nosey assistant this book would have never made it to print.

For all your support in those stressful times of fitting in working, cleaning, writing and worrying. For understanding the highs and lows my thanks go out to my girlfriend who has in-between her own lifestyle, health, family issues and affairs has been with me at the source of my journey from day one.

Thanks to

Friends and family.

Everything I have been given,
Everything I have achieved,
All my encouragement, support, love and care,
Every piece of me and what I have been blessed with is all down to the people who have never given up on my ideas, thoughts and incredible imagination. I have been so fortunate to have the continuous privilege of being led by example,

Thank you

Mum, Dad and Brother

I love you.

All characters in this book are purely fictional.